Praise for *The Reconnection*

D0300804

*"Eric is an amazing man with the superb gift of healing.
Read this book and be transformed!"*
— **John Edward,** psychic medium;
author of *Crossing Over* and *After Life*

"When I first received The Reconnection, *I sat down and read it
cover to cover in one evening. I was enthralled. It reads like a good
novel. But, unlike a novel, this book is the truth—the truth about a
revolutionary new way to heal and be healed that is available to anyone.
Filled with humor, insight, and the in-depth understanding and humility
that come only with the maturity of a good clinician and scientist,
Eric Pearl tells the story of how he became transformed by reconnective
energy, and how all of us can do the same. If you're serious
about health and healing, read this book!"*
— **Christiane Northrup, M.D.,** assistant clinical professor of OB/GYN,
University of Vermont College of Medicine; author of
Women's Bodies, Women's Wisdom and *The Wisdom of Menopause*

*"As a physician and a neuro-scientist, I have been trained to know
why and how a treatment works. When it comes to Reconnective
Healing, I don't know how it works. I simply know from personal
experience that it does. Eric Pearl's work has been a great gift for
me, and through this book, can be the same for you."*
— **Mona Lisa Schulz, M.D., Ph.D.,** author of *Awakening Intuition*

"This is a book that inspires the mind as it comforts the heart and celebrates the healing process. Dr. Pearl's vision of Reconnective Healing should be read by health-care professionals who wish to foster a higher level of healing in their patients and, in the process, heal themselves. The Reconnection should also be read by patients so they can not only heal themselves, but assist in the healing of others—and, through their example, they can inform their conventional physicians about contemporary energy medicine and the healing power of The Reconnection."
— **Gary E. R. Schwartz, Ph.D.,** and **Linda G. S. Russek, Ph.D.,** directors of the Human Energy Systems Laboratory at the University of Arizona; and authors of *The Living Energy Universe: A Fundamental Discovery That Transforms Science and Medicine*

"This is a wonderful book describing the evolution of a doctor-healer, told with wit, humor, and deep insights. Dr. Pearl's unique stories and experiences leading to the development of Reconnective Healing are both inspirational and moving. Eric Pearl has been given an unparalleled gift of healing, which he passes on to the rest of us. His approach to Reconnective Healing is simple, yet profound in its effects. It represents a new, nondirected form of energetic healing that goes beyond the formulas, techniques, and mantras that we have had to work with on this planet until now. I highly recommend it for health-care practitioners, as well as anyone else interested in awakening their own healing potential."
— **Richard Gerber, M.D.,** author of *Vibrational Medicine* and *Vibrational Medicine for the 21st Century*

"The Reconnection is a well-written, real-life story that could truly inspire people to follow their spiritual path and become healers."
— **Doreen Virtue, Ph.D.,** author of
The Lightworker's Way and *Healing with the Angels*

THE
RECONNECTION

HAY HOUSE TITLES OF RELATED INTEREST

BOOKS

THE INDIGO CHILDREN
The New Kids Have Arrived, by Lee Carroll and Jan Tober

THE LIGHTWORKER'S WAY
Awaken Your Spiritual Power to Know and Heal,
by Doreen Virtue, Ph.D.

YOUR SECRET LAWS OF POWER
The Modern Art of Healthy Living, by Alla Svirinskaya

YOU KNOW MORE THAN YOU THINK
How to Access Your Super-Subconscious Powers,
by Seka Nikolic

AUDIO PROGRAMS

DEVELOPING YOUR OWN PSYCHIC POWERS, by John Edward

All of the above are available at your local bookstore,
or may be ordered by visiting:

Hay House UK: www.hayhouse.co.uk
Hay House USA: www.hayhouse.com®
Hay House Australia: www.hayhouse.com.au
Hay House South Africa: www.hayhouse.co.za
Hay House India: www.hayhouse.co.in

THE
RECONNECTION

Heal Others,
Heal Yourself

DR. ERIC PEARL

HAY HOUSE, INC.
Australia • Canada • Hong Kong
South Africa • United Kingdom
United States

First published and distributed in the United Kingdom by:
Hay House UK Ltd, 292B Kensal Rd, London W10 5BE. Tel.: (44) 20 8962 1230;
Fax: (44) 20 8962 1239. www.hayhouse.co.uk

Published and distributed in the United States of America by:
Hay House, Inc., PO Box 5100, Carlsbad, CA 92018-5100. Tel.: (1) 760 431 7695 or
(800) 654 5126; Fax: (1) 760 431 6948 or (800) 650 5115.
www.hayhouse.com

Published and distributed in Australia by:
Hay House Australia Ltd, 18/36 Ralph St, Alexandria NSW 2015.
Tel.: (61) 2 9669 4299; Fax: (61) 2 9669 4144. www.hayhouse.com.au

Published and distributed in the Republic of South Africa by:
Hay House SA (Pty), Ltd, PO Box 990, Witkoppen 2068. Tel./Fax: (27) 11 467 8904.
www.hayhouse.co.za

Published and distributed in India by:
Hay House Publishers India, Muskaan Complex, Plot No.3, B-2, Vasant Kunj, New
Delhi – 110 070. Tel.: (91) 11 4176 1620; Fax: (91) 11 4176 1630.
www.hayhouse.co.in

Distributed in Canada by:
Raincoast, 9050 Shaughnessy St, Vancouver, BC V6P 6E5. Tel.: (1) 604 323 7100;
Fax: (1) 604 323 2600

Copyright © 2001 by Eric Pearl

Editorial supervision: Jill Kramer • Design: Summer McStravick

ISBN 978-1-4019-0210-0

Printed in the UK by CPI Group (UK) Ltd, Croydon, CR0 4YY.

❧ ❧ ❧

To my parents, for giving me life—
and for giving me the courage to live its truth.

To Aaron and Solomon, for giving me insight—
and for giving me the validation I needed to continue forward.

To God/Love/Universe, for giving.

❧ ❧ ❧

❧ CONTENTS ❧

❧ FOREWORD ❧

YOU ARE ABOUT TO READ a book about a courageous and caring clinician, Dr. Eric Pearl, who discovered that the key to health and healing is what he calls *The Reconnection*. When we first heard him speak at Dr. Andrew Weil's Program in Integrative Medicine at the University of Arizona, we were immediately impressed by Dr. Pearl's honesty and openness. Here was a man who was willing to give up one of the most lucrative chiropractic practices in Los Angeles to go on a spiritual healing journey to address some of the most important and controversial questions in contemporary medicine and healing.

Does energy, and the information it carries, play a central role in health and healing?

Can our minds connect with this energy, and can we learn to harness this energy to heal ourselves and others?

Is there a larger spiritual reality, comprised of living energy, which we can learn to connect with, that can not only promote our personal healing, but the healing of the planet as a whole?

We wondered, "Had Dr. Pearl lost his mind? Or, had he reconnected with the wisdom within his own heart and the living energy heart of the cosmos?"

The truth is, when we first met Dr. Pearl, we didn't know. However, Dr. Pearl was committed to "walking the talk." This included bringing his claims—and his talents—into a research laboratory whose motto is "If it is real, it will be revealed; and if it is fake, we'll catch the mistake."

The Human Energy Systems Laboratory at the University of Arizona is devoted to the integration of mind-body medicine, energy medicine, and spiritual medicine. Our purpose in working with Dr. Pearl was not to prove that Reconnective Healing works, but rather to give the Reconnective Healing process the opportunity to prove itself.

An Historic Connection to Reconnection

My [Gary's] personal relationship with the concept of reconnection goes back to my graduate Ph.D. program at Harvard University in the late 1960s. I was introduced to seminal research on self-regulation and healing conducted by one of the most integrative scientist-physicians in the first third of the last century.

In 1932, Professor Walter B. Cannon of Harvard University published his classic book, *The Wisdom of the Body*. Dr. Cannon described how the body maintained its physiological health—from the Greek *hael,* which means "wholeness"—through a process he termed "homeostasis." According to Cannon, the capacity of the body to maintain its homeostatic wholeness requires that feedback processes throughout the body be connected, and that the information traveling along this feedback highway network be fluid and accurate.

For example, if you connect a thermostat to a furnace so that whenever the temperature in your room goes below the level you set on the thermostat, the signal from the thermostat turns the furnace on, and vice versa, the temperature in your room will be maintained. The thermostat provides the feedback; the result is homeostasis between you and your room.

What makes all this work are the proper connections within the system. If you disconnect the feedback, the temperature will not be maintained. This, in a word, is the idea of feedback connection.

As a young assistant professor in the Department of Psychology and Social Relations at Harvard University, I derived the logic that led to the discovery that feedback connections are fundamental not only to physiological health and wholeness, but to health and wholeness at all levels in nature. The connection of feedback is fundamental to wholeness—be it energetic, physical, emotional, mental, social, global, and yes, even astrophysical.

I proposed that Cannon's "the wisdom of the body" might reflect a larger, universal principle. I called this "the wisdom of a system" or more simply, "the wisdom of connection":

When things are connected—be they

1. oxygen connected to hydrogen by chemical bonds in water;

2. the brain connected to physiological organs by neural, hormonal, or electromagnetic mechanisms in the body; or

3. the sun connected to earth by gravity and electromagnetic influences in the solar system . . .

. . . and information and energy circulates freely, any system has the capacity to be healthy, remain whole, and evolve.

When I was a professor of psychology and psychiatry at Yale University in the mid-'70s through the late '80s, I published scientific papers that applied this universal connection principle not only to mind-body wholeness and healing, but to wholeness and healing at all levels in nature (e.g., Schwartz, 1977; 1984). My colleagues and I proposed that there were five basic steps to achieving wholeness and healing: *attention, connection, self-regulation, order,* and *ease.*

Step 1: Voluntary *attention.* This is as simple as just experiencing your body, and the energy flowing within your body and between you and your environment.

Step 2: Attention creates *connection.* When you allow your mind, consciously or unconsciously, to experience energy and information, this process promotes connections not only within your body, but between your body and the environment.

Step 3: Connection fosters *self-regulation.* Like a team of athletes or musicians who together achieve greatness in sports or jazz, the dynamic connections among the players enables the team to organize and control itself (termed "self-regulation"), with the guiding assistance of coaches and conductors.

Step 4: Self-regulation promotes *order*. What you experience
as wholeness, success, or even beauty, reflects an
organizing process made possible by connections
allowing self-regulation.

Step 5: The order is expressed with *ease*. When everything
is connected properly, and the parts (the players) are
allowed to fulfill their respective roles, the self-regulation process can occur effortlessly. The process flows.

The reverse is also true. There are five basic steps to achieving disin-
tegration and disease: *disattention, disconnection, disregulation, disorder,*
and *disease.*

If you *disattend* to your body (Step 1), this creates a *disconnection* within
your body and between your body and the environment (Step 2), promot-
ing *disregulation* in the body (Step 3), which would be measured as *disorder* in the system (Step 4), and be experienced as *disease* (Step 5).

In a word, *connection* leads to *order* and *ease; disconnection* leads to
disorder and *disease.*

As you read Dr. Pearl's book, you will see these connecting steps come
to life at all levels—from the energetic, through mind-body, to the spiritual. The key to understanding this new level of healing is the prefix "re"
—*re*attending, *re*connecting, *re*-regulating, *re*ordering healing.

Discovering the Wisdom of Reconnection

In Stephen Sondheim's musical *Sunday in the Park with George,* which
is about the pointillist painter, George Seurat, the creation of beauty was
described as a connection process. Seurat was a master at organizing and
connecting colored dots, creating beautiful images that humble us to this
day. Sondheim reminds us of the importance of this process with his simple lyrics: "Connect, George, connect."

In the process of reading this book, you will take part in a connective
healing journey. Your mind and heart will be extended and united as
Dr. Pearl connects the dots of his life. You will enter the soul of a gifted
healer who has experienced personal doubts and pain as he discovered the
reconnection process, and you will witness the deep blessings and satisfaction he experienced as he saw his patients heal.

We do not wish to imply that everything written in this book is scientifically recognized. However, neither does Dr. Pearl. He shares his experiences, offers *his* conclusions, then lets *you* come to your own conclusions. The journey continues.

Dr. Pearl has a long-term commitment to evidence-based medicine. The basic science studies conducted in our laboratory to date are surprisingly consistent with his predictions, and future clinical studies are planned. As our book *The Living Energy Universe* suggests, wisdom for healing may be all around us, waiting to be tapped so that it may serve its highest purposes.

May you be as enlightened and inspired by this book as we have.

— **Gary E. R. Schwartz, Ph.D.,** and **Linda G. S. Russek, Ph.D.**

✎ ✎ ✎

Gary E. R. Schwartz, Ph.D., is a professor of psychology, medicine, neurology, psychiatry, and surgery; and director of the Human Energy Systems Laboratory at the University of Arizona. He is also vice-president for research and education in the Living Energy Universe Foundation. He received his Ph.D. from Harvard University in 1971, and was an assistant professor of psychology at Harvard until 1976. He was a professor of psychology and psychiatry at Yale University, director of the Yale Psychophysiology Center, and co-director of the Yale Behavioral Medicine Clinic until 1988.

Linda G. S. Russek, Ph.D., is clinical assistant professor of medicine and co-director of the Human Energy Systems Laboratory at the University of Arizona. She is also president of the Living Energy Universe Foundation and directs the *Celebrating the Living Soul* conference series (**www.livingenergyuniverse.com**).

✤ ✤ ✤

❧ PREFACE ❧

*"Everyone has a purpose in life . . . a unique gift or
special talent to give to others. And when we blend this unique
talent with service to others, we experience the ecstasy and exultation
of our own spirit, which is the ultimate goal of all goals."*
— Deepak Chopra, M.D.

I'VE BEEN GIVEN many wonderful gifts in my life. One of them is the amazing ability to bring forth healings—which, you will see as you turn these pages, I don't fully understand (although I'm getting closer). A second gift has been my discovery that there truly are worlds that exist outside of this one. A third gift is the opportunity I've been given to write this book and share the information I've acquired so far.

What's so wonderful about the first gift is that, through it, I realized that I had a purpose in life and that I've been blessed to not only be able to *recognize* that purpose, but to be living it actively and consciously. Of life's gifts, this is truly one of the highest.

The second gift gave me the ability to recognize my true *Self*—to understand that I am a spiritual being, and that my human experience is just that: my *human* experience. It is but *one* experience of who I am. There are others. As I see my spirit come forward in everything I do, I am able to see it—and touch it—in others as well. This is an amazing gift, and although it's been right in front of me the whole time, I'd never even noticed it until now. This second gift gave me perspective on my purpose.

The third gift is the one that breathed a new element of life into the first two. I had, up until recently, only been sharing the gift of healing with others, one-person-at-a-time. Although I loved what I was doing, I knew it was to be shared with more people. I wasn't doing it a favor by keeping it to myself . . . and I wasn't keeping it to myself intentionally. I saw it as a gift (which it is), and therefore thought it couldn't be given by me to others (which it can).

It was patient with me. It knew that I would soon recognize the bigger picture. As its ability to entrain in others made itself known, I started giving seminars where larger numbers of people were able to interact with it firsthand. Discovering that this gift of healing can be activated in others via television was very exciting as well. As for the written word—well, that seems to bring a whole new dimension to its conveyance. What's so compelling about communicating via the print and broadcast media is that it enables so many more people to experience the activation of this healing ability in themselves. It was time, I realized, for a shift in our understanding; for the human race to see that—and I don't want to sound overly religious—wherever two or more are gathered, we may be of service to one another. We may facilitate another's healing. And now we may do so on levels never before available to us.

I came to realize that my gift was not only to help *others*, but to help *others* help others. This gave me an expanded vehicle with which to begin to fulfill my purpose.

This book is a combination of the instruction manual I was never given . . . and an activation to start you on your way.

If it is your intention either to *become* a healer, to take your current ability as a healer to greater levels—or simply to touch the stars to know that they really do exist—then this book was written for you.

But it was written for me as well. It is an expression of my purpose in life, which I finally found. Or, maybe I should say, my purpose found me. I hope that it helps you find yours as well.

— **Dr. Eric Pearl**

❧ ❧ ❧

❧ ACKNOWLEDGEMENTS ❧

I'D LIKE TO ACKNOWLEDGE:

Sonny and Lois Pearl, my parents, for their support of me in all ways.

Chad Edwards, whose integrity, ceaseless energy, and unwavering commitment to truth saved this book.

Hobie Dodd, whose extraordinary love, loyalty, friendship, and belief—as well as his ability to take care of my personal and business life—enabled me to create the time to sit down and write this book.

Jill Kramer, whose editing found the essence in my book, and made sure that others were able to find it as well.

Robin Pearl-Smith, my sister, for maintaining my Website, ceaselessly editing this book (along with my parents, Hobie, and Chad—before Jill got it), and helping to bring an understanding of The Reconnection into the world.

John Edward, for all his behind-the-scenes support.

Lorane, Harry, and Cameron Gordon, who opened their hearts to me and gave me my family-away-from-family and my home-away-from-home, helping me to be all that I could be.

Lee and Patti Carroll, whose friendship and belief helped sustain me through the process of writing this book.

John Altschul, who politely tried to ignore this until he had his own healing.

Aaron and Solomon, for their unworldly understanding.

Fred Ponzlov, for selflessly giving of himself and his time.

Mary Kay Adams, for her resolute support and encouragement.

Gary Schwartz and Linda Russek, for their time and energy invested in the research and documentation of Reconnective Healing, and for their beautiful Foreword to this book.

Reid Tracy, for his handling of this book and for treating me with kindness and respect.

The entire Hay House staff, including Tonya, Jacqui, Jenny, Summer, and Christy, for being there and beautifully coming through for this book whenever called upon.

Susan Shoemaker, who steeped countless cups of tea while reading this entire book aloud to me—*twice!*

Joel Carpenter, who allowed me into his home and always made sure I stopped writing long enough to eat.

Steven Wolfe, for being a grounding and stabilizing element in my life.

Craig Pearl, my brother, for not laughing.

And to God, the only One in this book
Who doesn't care how I spell His or Her name.

❧❧ ❧❧ ❧❧

PART I

❧❧

The Gift

*"How much longer will you
go on letting your energy sleep?
How much longer are you going to stay
oblivious of the immensity of yourself?"*
— from *A Cup of Tea,*
by Bhagwan Shree Rajneesh

❧ CHAPTER ONE ❧

First Steps

*"There are only two ways to live your life. One is as though
nothing is a miracle. The other is as though everything is a miracle."*
— Albert Einstein

The Miracle of Gary

How did this person ever get up the steps? I thought, looking through
the picture window beside the entrance to my office. My new patient
was just reaching the top of the staircase. He moved in a series of
one-step lunges interspersed with pauses, during which he stared down at
the next step, preparing himself for the effort. Once again I wondered if
starting a chiropractic practice on the second floor of a building with no
elevator had been the best course of action. Wasn't it sort of like opening
a brake repair shop at the bottom of a steep hill?

I didn't have many options at the time I went into practice in 1981,
and, as it appeared, I had even fewer now . . . although the reasons had
changed. During my 12 years here, my chiropractic practice had grown into
one of the largest in the city of Los Angeles. How could I just pull up and
relocate?

I decided not to go out and help this man make it up the last couple of
steps. I didn't want to diminish his imminent sense of accomplishment. I
could see in his face the resolute determination of a mountain climber scal-
ing the final slope of Mount Everest. As he lurched onto the landing at last,
I couldn't help but be reminded of the dauntless climb up the bell tower
by the Hunchback of Notre Dame.

A glance at the patient's paperwork revealed that his name was Gary.

He had come to me due to his lifelong back pain. This wasn't surprising. Although young and healthy, he had a tortured posture that became evident the moment his body came into view. His right leg was several inches shorter than his left, and his right hip was much higher in placement. Due to his deformity, he walked with an exaggerated limp, swinging his right hip outward with each step, then thrusting his body forward to catch up. His right foot turned inward and rested atop his left so that his two legs acted as one larger leg, balancing the weight of his upper body. To keep from falling, his back would hunch forward at approximately a 30-degree angle, giving the appearance that he was readying himself to dive into a pool. His posture and gait resulted in his intense back problems, from childhood up to the present.

Soon, Gary was filling me in on his history. It turned out that, in a way, he'd been struggling up a staircase from the moment of his birth. The doctor had cut his umbilical cord too soon, interrupting the supply of oxygen to his infant brain. By the time his lungs took over, the damage was done: His brain was affected in such a way that the right side of his body failed to develop symmetrically.

By the age of 14, Gary explained, he had visited more than 20 doctors in an attempt to remedy his condition. Surgery was performed to help his gait and posture by elongating the Achilles tendon on his right heel. It didn't work. He was given orthopedic shoes and leg braces. No improvement. When the spasms that plagued his right leg became more and more violent, Gary was prescribed powerful antispasmodic drugs. The spasms seemed to thrive on the medication, which otherwise dulled and disoriented him.

Finally, Gary found himself in the office of a famous and highly regarded specialist. If anyone could help him, Gary was sure that this was the man.

After a detailed examination, the doctor sat down, looked him in the eyes, and told him that there was nothing he could do. Gary would always have back problems, he said, adding that his problems would increase with age, his skeleton would continue to deteriorate, and he would eventually spend his life confined to a wheelchair. Gary had just stared at the doctor.

Gary had pinned all his hopes and expectations on this medical professional, but he left that office feeling more dejected than ever. That was the day, as Gary tells it, that he "mentally wrote off the medical establishment."

Thirteen years passed. While working out with an acquaintance, Gary happened to mention to her that he'd been experiencing some unusually severe back pain. Oddly enough, she'd been a patient of mine two years earlier following a serious motorcycle accident. She referred Gary to my office.

So here he was.

Absorbed in his history, I looked up from taking my notes and asked, "Do you know what goes on here?"

Gary looked at me, somewhat puzzled by the question. "You're a chiropractor, right?"

I nodded *yes*, consciously deciding not to say more. There was an expectant feeling in the air. Was I the only one who felt it?

Bringing Gary into a different room, I placed him on a table and adjusted his neck. Instructing him to return in 48 hours for reevaluation, I informed him that the initial visit was over.

Two days later, Gary returned.

As before, I had him lie on the table. The adjustment took only a few seconds. This time I asked him to relax and close his eyes . . . and not to open them until I asked him to do so. I brought my hands, palms down, about a foot or so in the air over his torso, slowly noting the various yet still unusual sensations I was feeling as I brought my hands farther up toward his head. Turning my palms inward, I continued bringing them up until they were each facing one of his temples. As I held them there, I watched Gary's eyes dart back and forth, rapidly and with strength, side-to-side, with an intensity that indicated that he was anything but asleep.

I was instinctively drawn to bring my hands down to the area of Gary's feet. I held my palms gently facing his soles. My hands felt as if they were suspended by an invisible support structure. Due to Gary's birth deformity, his right leg remained in its inwardly rotated position even when he was lying on his back. As I watched the bottoms of his stockinged feet, I had no idea what I was about to witness. It was as if his feet came to life. Not just alive as all of our feet are alive, but as if they became two distinct living entities, distinct from one another—and distinctly *not* Gary. In spellbound fascination, I observed the motions of his feet. An independent consciousness almost seemed present in each.

Suddenly, Gary's right foot began a movement pattern akin to lightly "pumping" a gas pedal. As this "pumping" continued, a second movement was added—an outward rotational motion that took his right foot from its original position of resting atop the left, to a toes-up position, one that had the toes pointing up toward the ceiling just as they were on his left foot. Not aware if I were still breathing, I stared in silence while Gary's eyes continued to dart like a speeding metronome on a grand piano. Then his foot, still pumping, rotated back and settled into its original position. The pattern repeated. Out. In. Out. In. Then it seemed to stop. I waited. And waited. And waited. Nothing further seemed to be forthcoming.

I found myself walking alongside the table until I was standing by Gary's right side. Although it had not been my pattern to touch a person's body when I did this, I found myself compelled to very lightly rest my hands on his right hip, my right hand on top of my left, yet not directly one over the other. I looked down toward Gary's feet. Again, the right foot began to move, first in the pumping fashion, then it resumed its rotation. Out. In. Out. In. Out.

I waited. And I waited. Nothing more seemed to occur.

I removed my hands from Gary's hip, then gently, with two fingers, touched Gary on his chest. "Gary? I think we're finished."

Gary's eyes were still darting about, although I could see that he was trying to open them. Approximately 30 seconds later, when they did open, Gary looked a little dazed. "My foot was moving," he told me, as if I hadn't seen it. "I could feel it, but I couldn't stop it. I felt really hot all over, then I felt some kind of energy building up in my right calf. Then . . . you'll think this is crazy, but it felt as if invisible hands were turning my foot, yet it didn't feel like hands at all."

"You can stand up now," I said, doing my best not to appear nonplused, yet still trying to take it all in myself. Gary stood up—for the first time in his 26 years—six feet tall, with two independent legs.

I watched in grateful amazement as Gary stood there: His spine was straight, and his hips were level and balanced. His expression began to reflect his own understanding of what had just happened. As he took a couple of tentative steps, I could tell that a bit of the limp remained, but nothing like the lurching leg-swing of before. Not even close.

Gary left my office with an enormous smile on his face, and I watched him walk gracefully down the steps.

Signposts

On that day, energy had clearly risen to an entirely new level. Why? I couldn't say. It would simply rise to new levels, sometimes every week, sometimes every few days, sometimes several times in a given day. Even then, I knew that although the energy came *through* me, I didn't create or even direct it. Someone else was doing that, someone more powerful than I. Although I'd been doing a lot of reading lately, what was happening to me didn't fit in with any of the "energy healing" I'd learned about in these books. This was more than simply "energy." This carried with it life and intelligence beyond the many "techniques" that fill bookshelves and New Age periodicals. This was something different. This was something very real.

What happened that afternoon with Gary didn't just change *his* life, but it was about to change mine as well. Not that Gary was the only patient I'd worked with in this fashion—moving my hands above their bodies. That had been going on for over a year. Nor was he the only patient who had received a remarkable healing during the experience. However, he did represent the most extreme case by far—the patient who had started out with the most severe disability and who had walked out of my office with the most striking and obvious results. Almost two dozen of the finest physicians in the country had been unable to correct—or even improve—Gary's gait, posture, or the rotation in his hip and leg, yet this anomaly, and its associated pain, were virtually gone. In a matter of minutes. Gone.

I once again wondered why this energy had chosen to make its appearance through *me*. I mean, if I were sitting on a cloud scouring the planet for just the right person upon whom I could bestow one of the rarest and most sought-after gifts in the universe, I don't know whether I would have reached through the ethers, pointed my finger through the vast multitudes of people, and said, "Him! That's the one. Give this gift to him."

Now maybe it didn't happen in quite that way, but that's the way it felt to me.

I certainly hadn't spent my life sitting around on a mountaintop in Tibet, contemplating my navel and eating bowls of dirt with chopsticks. I'd spent 12 years building my practice, and I had three homes, a Mercedes, two dogs, and two cats. I was a man who occasionally overindulged, watched more TV than a 12-year-old couch potato, and thought I was doing everything I was "supposed" to be doing. Oh, I'd had my share of problems—in fact, they'd built to a climax just before all these bizarre events started to occur—but, in general, my life was proceeding according to plan.

But *whose* plan? That was the question I now had to ask myself. Because when I looked back, I could see that there had been certain signposts along the road of my life—strange occurrences, coincidences, and events—which, although they didn't amount to much individually . . . collectively, and with the advantage of hindsight, suggested that I'd never really been walking along the road I thought I'd chosen.

Where was the first signpost? How far back did the evidence go? If you asked my mother, it went all the way back to the day I was delivered from her womb. My birth had been, in her words, "unusual." Of course, most mothers remember their first birthing experience as special and unique. But it's not the same thing. Some women go through days of torturous labor. Others give birth in the woods or in the back seat of a taxi. My mother? She died on the delivery table while in labor with me.

But dying wasn't what bothered her. What bothered her was having to come back to life.

✌ ✌ ✌

❧ CHAPTER TWO ❧

Lessons from Life After Death

*"There is a logical reason for everything that is happening
in this world and beyond—and it all makes perfect sense.
One day, you will understand the divine purpose of God's plan."*
— Lois Pearl

The Hospital

When will this baby be born? she agonized. In the labor room, Lois
Pearl, my mother, had been doing her breathing exercises and bearing down, bearing down . . . but nothing was happening. No baby.
No dilation. Just pain and more pain, and the doctor popping in to check on
her between delivering other babies. She tried not to cry out; she was determined not to make a scene. After all, this was a hospital. There were sick
people here.

Still, the next time the doctor came around, my mother looked up at
her pleadingly, and with tears streaming, asked, "Is this ever going to end?"

Concerned, the doctor placed one hand firmly on my mother's abdomen
to see if I had "dropped" enough to be delivered. The doctor's face showed
that she wasn't quite convinced that I had done so. But taking into account
my mother's excruciating pain, the doctor turned toward the nurse and reluctantly said, "Take her in."

My mother was placed on a gurney and wheeled into the delivery room.
As the doctor continued to press on her abdomen, my mother noticed that
the room was suddenly filled with the sound of someone screaming very
loudly. *Boy,* she thought, *that woman's making a real fool of herself!* Then
she realized that she and the medical personnel were the only ones in the
room—which meant that the screaming must be coming from her. She was

making a scene, after all. That really bothered her.

"*When* is this going to end?"

The doctor gave her a comforting look and a short whiff of ether. It was like placing a Band-Aid on a severed limb.

"*We're losing her . . .*"

My mother could barely hear the voice over the roar of motors—huge motors, like something you'd find in a factory, not a hospital. They hadn't started off that loudly. The sound, accompanied by a tingling sensation, had begun around the soles of her feet. Then it began climbing up her body as if the motors were moving upward, getting louder and louder as they progressed, shutting off the feeling in one area before they moved to the next. Only numbness was left in their wake.

Above the sound of the motors, the pain of labor continued with glaring intensity.

My mother knew that she'd remember that pain for the rest of her life. Her female ob-gyn—a practical, no-nonsense, country-style M.D.—believed that women should experience the "full expression" of childbirth. Which meant no painkillers. Not even during delivery, unless you counted the merest whiff of ether at the peak of contraction.

Strangely, none of the doctors or nurses appeared distracted. Here was this thundering sound, yet nobody in the delivery room seemed to notice it. My mother wondered, *How can this be?*

So the motors, and the numbness they left behind, should have been a relief. But as they rumbled past my mother's pelvis to her waist, she was struck by what she knew would happen when they reached her heart.

We're losing her . . .

No! She was flooded with a sense of resistance. Pain or no pain, she didn't want to die—she imagined the people she loved in mourning. But no matter how she struggled, the motors would not reverse. They proceeded upward, numbing her an inch at a time, as if erasing her existence. She was powerless to stop them. As my mother came to this realization, something strange happened. Although she still didn't *want* to die, suddenly a peace fell over her.

Losing her . . .

The motors reached her sternum. Their roar filled her head.

And then she began to *rise. . . .*

The Journey

It wasn't my mother's *body* that was rising into the air. It was what she could only think of as her *soul*. She was being drawn upward, gravitating purposefully *toward* something. She didn't look back. No longer conscious of her physical surroundings, she knew that she'd already left the delivery room and its motors behind. She kept rising, moving upward. And, although she had no conscious knowledge of life after death, or of anything "spiritual," for that matter, it was of little consequence. It doesn't require a spiritual background to recognize when your fundamental essence is leaving your body and beginning to rise. There can only be one explanation for that.

My mother's final realization from the delivery table was that, although she was leaving everything that was familiar behind, *she no longer minded.* This surprised her initially. As soon as she stopped fighting and "let go," her journey began. What came to her first was a feeling of overall peace, tranquility, and absence of all worldly responsibilities. None of the worrisome details of everyday life to bog her down. No deadlines to meet, no mundane tasks to accomplish, no expectations to be met, no limits to be set. *No more fears of the unknown.* One by one, they were all melting away . . . and what a relief it was. What a *great* relief. As this was happening, a lighter feeling was coming over her, and she became aware of the fact that she was *floating.* She was feeling so light, with the melting away of all of these worldly responsibilities, that she rose to an even higher level. And so began my mother's ascent, only stopping to absorb knowledge of one kind or another.

She rose through a succession of different levels—she doesn't recall a distinct "tunnel," as some who have had similar experiences have reported. What she did recall was that along the way she encountered "others." These were more than just "people." They were "beings," "spirits," "souls" of those whose time had ended here on Earth. These "souls" spoke with her, although *spoke* may not be the most accurate word. The communication was nonverbal, a kind of thought transference that left no doubt as to what was being conveyed. Doubt did not exist here.

My mother learned that verbal language, as we know it, is not so much an *assistance* to communication as it is a communication *barrier.* It's one of the hurdles we are given to master as part of our learning experience here on Earth. It's also part of what keeps us in the limited scope of understanding in which we are to function in order to gain mastery of our other lessons.

The soul—the "core" of a person— is the only thing that survives or matters, my mother realized. Souls exhibit their natures clearly. There were no faces, no bodies, and nothing to hide behind, yet she recognized each for exactly who they were. Their physical facade was no longer a part of them. It was left behind as a remembrance of the role they once played in the lives of their loved ones, to be enshrined in the memory of their existence. This testament to the truth of their former physical being is all that remains here on Earth. Their true essence had transcended.

My mother learned how unimportant our exterior appearance and physical mannerisms actually are, and how shallow our attachment to their value is. Her lesson to learn on that level was to neither judge people by appearance—including race or color—nor by their creed or level of education. It was to discover who they really *are*, to see what's inside, to get past the exterior and behold their real identity. And, although this was a lesson she already knew *here*, somehow the illumination gained *there* was infinitely more intricate, infinitely more expansive.

It was impossible to judge the passage of time. My mother knew that she was there long enough to rise through all the levels. She also knew that each of the levels taught different lessons.

The first level was that of Earthbound souls—those who are not ready to leave. These are the ones having a difficult time separating themselves from the familiar. They are usually spirits who feel they have unfinished business to attend to. They may have left sick or handicapped loved ones whose care was their responsibility (and they are reluctant to desert them), lingering on this first level until they feel able to release themselves from their Earthly bonds. Or, they may have met a sudden or violent death that didn't allow them the time to understand that they had died, as well as the process they would have to go through to follow the path of ascension. Either way, they still feel strong ties to the living and are just not ready to let go. Until they come to the realization that they can no longer function on that plane, that they no longer belong there, and that they are no longer of that dimension, they will remain on the first level— the closest to their former life.

My mother's memories from the second level seem somewhat vague, yet her memories from the third are quite vivid.

When she rose to the third level, she remembers experiencing a heavy feeling. She felt a sadness when she realized that this was the level of those who had taken their own lives. These souls were now in limbo. They seemed to have been isolated, moving neither up nor down. They had no direction.

There was an aimless quality to their presence. Would they be allowed to ascend at some point in order to complete their lesson and evolve in their development? She couldn't comprehend that they would not. Maybe it was just taking them longer, but this, she felt, was pure speculation. This was not an answer my mother was able to bring back. Whatever the case, these souls were not at rest—and experiencing this level was very unpleasant, not only for those spending their time there, but for those passing through as well. The lesson from this, the third level, was indelible and clear: *Taking your own life interrupts God's plan.*

Additional Lessons

There were other lessons my mother was able to bring back as well. She was shown the futility of mourning for those who have died. If there was one regret experienced by the spirits who had passed, it was the pain suffered by those they left behind. They want us to rejoice in their passing, to "trumpet them home," because when we die, we are where we want to be. Our grieving is for *our* loss, the loss of the place in our lives once occupied by that person. Their existence, whether experienced as pleasant or unpleasant, was part of our learning process. When they die, we lose that lesson's "source." Hopefully, we had either learned what we were to have learned, or, by reflecting upon their life as it had intermingled with ours, we would eventually be able to do so. She knew that the passage of time—from when we leave heaven to go through our lives here on Earth, to when we return—is but a snap of the fingers in our eternal consciousness, and that we will all be together "momentarily." It is then that we realize that this is how it was meant to be.

She was also shown that, no matter what seemingly terrible or unfair things happen to people here on Earth, *it is not God's fault.* When innocent children are killed, good people die after prolonged illnesses, or someone is injured or disfigured, it has nothing to do with *blame* or *fault.* These are *our* lessons to learn—the ones in *our* divine plan—and we've agreed to carry them out. They are lessons for our evolution—for both the givers and the receivers.

In the larger picture, *these occurrences are under the direction and control of the person experiencing them.* The action, or the playing out of it, is merely our orchestration of events. Understanding this, she could see how inappropriate it is to question how God could let such things happen, or, based upon these events, to question whether God exists at all. My mother now understood that there was a perfectly logical explanation for it all. It was *so* perfect that she wondered why she hadn't known it all along. And somehow, seeing the whole picture, she realized that everything—*everything*—is as it should be.

My mother also learned that war is a temporary state of barbarism— an ignorant and inept way of settling differences, and at some point, it will no longer exist. These souls find humanity's addiction to warfare not just primitive, but ridiculous—young men being sent out to fight old men's battles for the acquisition of land. One day, humankind will look back on the whole concept and ask, *Why?* When there are enough evolved souls with vast intelligence to solve problems, there will be an end to war altogether.

My mother even found out why people who, to all appearances, had done "horrible" things in life were received there without judgment. Their actions became lessons from which they were to learn, and from which they were to become more perfect beings. They were to evolve from the level of their choices. Of course, they would have to come back to Earth again and again until they absorbed the knowledge derived from the far-reaching consequences of their behavior. They would go through this cycle of birth and rebirth for as long as it took them to evolve and finally return Home.

✎ ✎ ✎

When the lessons were complete, my mother ascended to the top level. Once there, she stopped rising and began gliding effortlessly forward, drawn steadily and purposefully toward some kind of force. The most beautiful colors and shapes whirled past her on either side. They were like landscapes, except . . . there was no land. Somehow she knew that they were flowers and trees, yet they were in no way like anything here on Earth. These unique, indescribable hues and forms that didn't exist in the world she'd left behind filled her with wonder.

Gradually, my mother became aware that she was skimming above a kind of road, a lane lined on either side by familiar souls—friends, relatives, and people she knew from many lifetimes. They had come to receive her, to guide her and let her know that everything was okay. It was an indescribable feeling of peace and bliss.

At the far end of the road, my mother saw a light. It was like the sun, so bright that she was afraid it would burn her eyes. Yet the beauty of it was dazzling. She couldn't turn her eyes away. Surprisingly, even as she drew closer, her eyes felt no pain. The exquisite glow of the light seemed familiar—somehow comfortable. She found herself surrounded by its corona and knew that the light was much more than just a radiance: It was the core of the Supreme Being. She had reached the level of the all-knowing, all-consuming, all-accepting, and all-loving Light. My mother knew she was *Home*. This was where she belonged. This was where she had come from.

Then, the Light communicated with her without words. With a non-verbal thought or two, it conveyed enough information to fill volumes. It spread her lifetime—*this* lifetime—out before her in pictures. It was wonderful to see; almost everything she'd ever said or done was displayed in plain sight. She could actually feel the pain or joy she'd given others. Through this process, she was receiving her lessons—*without any judgment*. However, although there was no judgment, *she* knew it was a good life.

After a while, my mother was given the knowledge that she was being sent back. But she didn't *want* to go. Funny, in spite of all the struggle she'd put up against dying in the first place, she really didn't want to leave at all now. She was so beautifully at peace—ensconced in her new surroundings, her new understandings, her old friends. She wanted to stay for eternity. How could anyone expect her to leave?

In answer to these silent pleas, my mother was made to understand that she had not finished her job back on Earth: She had to return to raise her child. Part of the reason she had been brought here was to acquire special insight into how to do just that!

Suddenly, my mother felt herself being drawn out from the core of the Light and back along the path that she had previously traveled. But now she was going in the opposite direction, and she knew she was returning to her life on Earth. Leaving the familiar souls, the colors and shapes, and the Light Itself, made her feel a deep yearning and sadness.

As she receded from the Light, my mother's knowledge began slipping away. She knew that she'd been *programmed* to forget; she wasn't *supposed* to remember. She tried desperately to cling to what was left, knowing that this was definitely not a dream. She struggled to hang on to the memories and impressions, many of which were gone already, and she felt a terrible loss. However, she felt an inner peace, now instilled with the knowledge that when it was her time to return Home, she would be welcomed with love. This, she knew she would remember. She no longer feared death.

At that moment, my mother heard the distant sound of motors. This time they started at the top of her head and began to work their way down. Beyond the roar, she began to hear voices—human voices—and then the beating of her own heart.

Most of the pain, she noticed, was gone.

The motors moved down, down, down . . . their roar fading in intensity. Soon there was nothing left of the motors but a tingling in the soles of her feet. And then not even that. It was over. She had returned to what people like to think of as the "real" world.

A very relieved-looking doctor leaned over her, smiling. "Congratulations, Lois," she said. "You have a beautiful baby boy."

The Meaning of It All

They hadn't shown me to my mother yet. First they had to clean me up, weigh me, and count my toes. So, it was on to her hospital room. As they wheeled my mother into the hallway, the total sense of what she'd experienced and absorbed suddenly overwhelmed her. She intuitively knew that she had already forgotten many of the insights which, only moments ago, were hers: why the sky was blue, why the grass was green, why the world was round, and how creation came about—the perfect logic of it all. Yet she also knew with certainty that there *is* a Supreme Being. There *is* a God.

There was also one realization that she brought back with unequivocal clarity: *"We are placed here to learn lessons that make us more complete souls. We have to live this plan out on this level before we're ready to go on to another level. That's why some people are old souls, while others are young ones."*

These days, you might be able to find a lot of this information in metaphysical books, but that wasn't true at the time. Bookstores didn't have New Age sections back then, and these lessons certainly weren't taught as part of our basic religious traditions. My mother didn't have friends who talked about these things, nor had she entered the hospital to seek enlightenment— she simply wanted to get a very reluctant fetus out of her body before she went insane from the pain!

There was no question that she *had* changed, however. She could feel it—and she knew that, ironically, part of that change was the result of having to leave the memories of so many lessons behind. All of her life she'd been compulsive, a perfectionist. Now, as she found herself yearning to embody every single one of the principles she'd been taught, she discovered that she couldn't remember most of them. How can you practice what you can't remember?

Therefore, my mother decided that it was time to go easier on herself . . . and others. That is, maybe she'd allow a bit of dust inside the house, not carry a bottle of Lysol on vacation trips to wipe down the insides of hotel room lavatories, and begin to accept things as they are.

As the gurney rolled down the corridor, my father appeared at my mother's side, keeping pace. She gestured for him to bend closer. "When we get back to the room," she whispered, "I have something to tell you that I've been programmed to forget."

When they were in the room together, alone except for a couple of women in hospital beds, my mother whispered, "Don't repeat anything I say, Sonny. People will think I'm crazy."

"I won't."

She went on to describe everything she could still remember, trying to save the few grains of sand that clung to her fingers. My father listened quietly, and she was certain that he didn't doubt a single word she said. He knew she would never make up such a crazy story.

When she was done, exhaustion began to pull her into sleep. She urged my father to go home and write everything down as soon as he could. This information was too precious to lose. He agreed.

Upon awakening, she found herself looking at the woman in the next bed. My mother recognized her from the previous day. Her first thought was a groggy, *Gee, is she ugly!* And then she said to herself, "Now wait a minute. You just experienced the realization that a person's appearance doesn't matter." The irony of it all made her laugh.

"You were talkin' all night when you got back from havin' the baby," the roommate said.

"I was?"

"You were recitin' Scripture."

"What did I say?"

"I don't know. You were speakin' in tongues."

Speaking in tongues? Mom didn't know any foreign or ancient languages; for that matter, she couldn't recite anything other than the 23rd Psalm—and only in English at that.

She lay back in bed. So many questions. If she'd had any doubts before about what had happened to her the previous day, she didn't now. Something very unusual had gone on in that delivery room. She knew it wasn't a dream, if only because dreams don't make you change, not in such a profound way. How could you go into a dream being afraid of death and come out not only unafraid, but actually at ease with it—and knowing that you'd *always* feel that way?!

My mother wanted to delve deeper into her experience. In particular, she wanted to know exactly what had been going on with her body in the delivery room while her consciousness was off communing with beings of pure light.

She soon discovered that finding out wasn't going to be so easy.

When my mother asked the doctor if anything "strange" had happened in the delivery room, she was told, "No, it was a normal delivery." According to the doctor, the only complication, a minor one at that, had been the necessity of using forceps to move the baby into proper birth position—a very common practice at the time.

Code of Silence

A normal delivery?

This couldn't be the truth. The phrase "normal delivery" didn't coincide with "We're losing her."

Next, my mother questioned the R.N.'s who had worked with her in either the labor or delivery rooms, but she couldn't get anyone to own up to remembering her speaking in tongues, nor admit to any problems at all.

"Everything went just fine," she was told.

If M.D.'s and R.N.'s were the only people present during the birthing process, that would probably have been the end of it. But eventually my mother remembered a practical nurse who had also been in the O.R. during my delivery. Practical nurses worked in the trenches. They went about their business quietly, efficiently, and without fanfare. They often went unnoticed and were almost always under-appreciated. *Practical nurses didn't have much reason to hide the truth when things went wrong.*

So, my mother confronted the practical nurse, saying, "I know something happened to me in that O.R."

After a long pause, the nurse shrugged. "I can't talk about it, but all I *can* tell you is, *you . . . were . . . lucky.*"

We're losing her?

You were lucky?

This was enough to confirm what my mother already knew: Something special *had* happened to her that day in the delivery room, something that went far beyond the joy of squeezing little me into the world without the benefit of anesthesia. The doctors *had*, in fact, lost her. She had died—and returned. In fact, she would come to think of what happened to her not as a "near-death" experience, but as a "life-after-death" experience. "Near-death" is a watered-down term. My mother hadn't been *near* death. She'd *died*. And like other people who have died and come back, she'd returned a different person. She now understood that whatever came her way in life, "good" or "bad," it would be exactly what her soul needed at that time in order to progress. "You *do* come back . . . until you get it right." It's part of the evolution.

This lesson turned out to be a very apt and timely one. She had just given birth to me, and in her eyes, I was out of the realm of the ordinary from the moment I was born.

𝒟 𝒟 𝒟

Was this a typical motherly overstatement? Perhaps, except that my mother insists that she saw some evidence that I was unusual the very first time she laid eyes on me, the day after my birth. I was the only newborn in the nursery, and as she walked in with a bottle of formula in her hand, she approached my bassinet and peered in. I was lying on my stomach, awake. "Hello, little stranger," she greeted. "It's you and me against the world. You and me."

At the sound of her voice, I raised myself up on my forearms, and elevating my bobbing head, I slowly turned to the left, then slowly back around to the right, as if to take in my new surroundings. My mother looked at this sight in wonderment. Could this be possible? She had always been told that a newborn's neck muscles were far too weak to do something like that.

My mother started to set the bottle on a nearby table, then hesitated. Who knew what germs might be on the table's surface? She could picture them swarming up the outside of the bottle through the opening in the nipple, contaminating the formula. But hadn't she also just learned that she was better off ignoring some of these petty obsessions that used to consume her—that there was a reason and a balance to everything?

Almost. My mother compromised by folding a tissue and putting it between the bottle and the tabletop as she reached down to pick me up. She'd fallen in love with me the moment she saw me.

Later, when the doctor came in to examine her, Mom told her about my lifting my head. The doctor said firmly, "They can't do that." Then she left to examine me in the nursery.

A second later, Mom heard the doctor's voice from the nursery in the next room. "Oh, pshaw," the doctor said, her voice almost scolding. "You're not supposed to be able to do that. . . ."

At that moment, my mother felt sure that something extraordinary was at work here.

❧ ❧ ❧

❧ CHAPTER THREE ❧

Childish Things

"Kids say the darndest things."
— Art Linkletter

A s a child, I'm told I learned quickly but was very easily bored. I was imaginative and moody, thoughtful and reckless, loving and selfish. Like most young children, I was convinced that the universe revolved around me and my needs. And why not? There were few boundaries in my mind between what I desired and what I expected to get. I believed that everything should go my way. Everything.

Including family planning.

My mother felt the first stirrings of new life in her womb around the time I turned two. The sensation came in the form of two distinct "flutterings," so she was convinced that she was carrying twins. A team of ob-gyns insisted she was wrong, even as her belly began to swell . . . and swell . . . and swell. She was a tall, slim woman. From the rear, you saw only her height and slender silhouette, but when she turned sideways, there appeared a profile so extreme you could have rested a tray comfortably on her belly.

I loved to come in and listen to the thumpings inside my mother's stomach. When I put my ear against her, things would become very active inside. This fascinated me.

Some months later, my mother was back in the delivery room, but this time she was given painkillers. She heard no motors and went on no odysseys.

"Bear down," the doctors told her through an almost-bearable haze, and she did, then fell asleep. In a little while, they woke her. "Congratulations, you've got a beautiful baby girl." Pleased (and drugged), she nodded and fell back asleep. A few minutes later they woke her again. "Bear down."

Okay, she thought, *I knew this was coming.* So once again she obliged.

The next thing she remembered hearing was, "Congratulations, you have a beautiful baby boy." Knowing it was over, she gave herself permission to slide into a deep sleep.

Soon they were waking her again. "Bear down."

"Not another one!"

They laughed. "No, no, this is for the afterbirth."

When the twins finally arrived home, she was surprised to find that her first-born child, me, looked less than pleased.

"What's the matter?" she asked.

"I didn't want them," I said.

"You said you did," she responded warmly.

"No, I didn't."

"You said you wanted a brother and a sister."

Legs parted, right fist planted firmly on my hip, I looked my mother in the eyes. "I said I wanted a brother *or* a sister. *Oorrrrr* a sister. Take one back."

Little did I know the difficulties I'd encounter adjusting to siblings sharing a space that had been only mine until now. This would be a major challenge (okay, lesson for growth) for years to come.

Open the Door

The thing about precocious behavior is this: Sometimes it's cute and sometimes it isn't. From a very early age, I had a problem dealing with authority, and an even greater problem dealing with boredom. It was a volatile combination. If there was some little crevice I knew I wasn't supposed to explore, there I would be. If there was something I shouldn't do, most likely I'd do it. In my mother's words, to keep myself occupied, I became ingenious with "tricks" and explanations. Surrendering to sleep was only a way to rejuvenate. And even then, I was afraid that while I slept I might miss something.

An example of one of my tricks involved my maternal grandmother, "Nana." One day not long after my brother and sister had been brought home, Nana came to the house to baby-sit. This afforded my mother a much-needed break. My brother and sister were in their cribs, and I was temporarily occupied with the TV. Three large aluminum pots, one filled with diapers, the others with bottles of formula, were boiling busily on the stove, and a load of laundry had just finished drying in the basement. Nana went down to retrieve the clothes. Hard-working, fast, and practical, Nana was trying to hurry because she knew it wasn't the wisest thing to leave me alone for long. Arms laden with warm, freshly dried and folded laundry neatly piled high, she started up the stairs. Peering over the top, she suddenly saw the basement door start to swing shut. She tried to hurry, but the door slammed before she could get there. The lock clicked.

Leaning against the door holding the stack of clothes, Nana freed one hand and tested the knob. It wouldn't turn. "Open the door, Eric," she said in a sweetly controlled voice.

In an even sweeter voice, I replied, "Unh-uh."

"Come on, now, open the door."

"Unh-uh."

Nana knew that sounding firm wouldn't work with me. But she was not about to be outsmarted by a toddler, however precocious—especially with three pots of water boiling away in one room and two infants sleeping in another. So she tried a different approach. "I bet you can't reach the doorknob," she said, playing on my stubbornness.

"Yes, I can."

"I'll bet you can't."

There was quiet.

Nana broke into a sweat. She could almost hear the sound of my brain whirring, testing the situation. But finally, as she'd hoped, I had to prove myself. I pushed on the doorknob a little. She heard it rattle softly.

"I bet you can't unlock it," she said.

"Yes, I can."

Once again came the sweetly disguised dare: "Bet you can't."

There was another long pause. The clothes were getting heavy in her arms. The lock mechanism consisted of a small knob that you pushed in and turned. It would make a tiny *click* if it were released, and Nana waited for the sound. She'd have to move fast. She didn't want to hurt me by opening the door too quickly, but this was likely to be her only chance.

I couldn't resist.

Click.

Nana quickly pushed against the door, and it swung open faster than she'd expected. Still-warm, freshly folded laundry flew all over the floor. I was knocked over before I could run. Shocked, I sat there crying.

Nana hurried to shut off the boiling water, then came over to comfort me.

I was only two and a half years old, and already, Nana knew that she had her baby-sitting career cut out for her.

In the Clouds

Nana was my mother's mother, and "Bubba" was my father's. Bubba was a warm, strong, old-world-style grandmother who would give those big, suctioning European cheek-kisses—the kind that would make a Hoover blush. She was full of life, with boundless energy and a risqué sense of humor, often embarrassing some of the more "conservative" relatives. She'd sit me next to her at the holiday dinners; and on overnight stays, she'd take me out into her yard in the morning to pick strawberries and other fruit, and then prepare a great big breakfast. Afterwards, she'd carry me around in one arm like a feather while she'd clean, dust, vacuum, and talk on the phone. I loved all that motion, that feeling of traveling through space without using my feet. More and faster, that's what I wanted. Boy, did I love her.

One January day, Bubba went into the hospital and never came out.

Apparently, while lying in her hospital bed, she felt a pain in her chest, reached for the nurse's call button—and didn't make it.

Now my parents had to deal with Bubba's sudden departure from my life.

"She went to sleep," they told me, "and won't wake up again."

I gave this some thought, then dismissed it. "I can wake her up," I said. "I bet if we put three aspirin in her mouth and I jump up and down on her belly, she'll wake up." The jumping up and down on her stomach was my additional strategy, something to assist in case the taste of aspirin dissolving on her tongue wasn't a sufficient inducement for her to open her eyes and resume life.

That was one of the few times I remember seeing my father cry.

The funeral was held shortly thereafter. I was not allowed to attend. My parents felt that, at age five, it would be too traumatic for me to see my grandmother's lifeless body. Bubba was gone, and everyone got to say good-bye but me.

At night I'd lie in bed and think about her. Sometimes I'd cry quietly.

I missed her, and although I didn't understand the concept at the time, I'd had no sense of *closure*.

Meanwhile, though, I knew that even if I hadn't been able to say my farewells to Bubba, she hadn't forgotten *me*. I knew exactly where she was, and I knew she watched over me just as she always had. I knew because she'd help me out when I "needed" it—like when I was playing outside the house with my friends and it started to rain. Everyone would want to go home and the game would end, so I'd tell them all: "Wait right there; I'll be right back." While everyone huddled under my porch overhang, I would run around to the side of the house where no one could see me. Then I'd look up at the sky and say, "Bubba, would you please make it stop raining?"

And more often than not, the rain would stop. It seemed that my Bubba hadn't really left me after all.

At Odds with School

The time soon came to start kindergarten. From the moment I walked in the door, school bored me half to death. Most of my time was spent day-dreaming, but not the typical fantasies of a young boy—playing ball, being a hero, fighting off monsters. (Well, sometimes I fought off a giant tornado or two . . . but doesn't everyone?) More often I imagined that I was the Oracle of Delphi. I didn't really know who or what the Oracle of Delphi was, yet somehow I pictured myself sitting in a far-off cave tending to hordes of people who traveled long distances to seek my counsel.

I also contemplated acts that I just *knew* could be performed, like passing my hands through walls. I was sure that if I could just lock myself in my bedroom for three days, I could figure out how to do this. Strangely enough, no one seemed to be willing to let me. They probably tried it when they were kids and decided that it was a waste of time.

If the teachers disapproved of my daydreaming, they probably disliked my lack of attentiveness even more. I was frequently disruptive: misbehaving and drawing attention to myself, or ignoring them and getting lost in my own world. Before my first year was up, I'd been in trouble so many times that my mother finally broke down crying in front of the school director.

"When is this ever going to end?" she sobbed, inadvertently echoing the words she'd used when I was born.

"When he gets interested in something," the director said.

"When does that happen?"

"It can happen at any time." The director paused, then gave a helpless laugh. "With *my* son, it wasn't until college."

It wasn't that I didn't have interests; they just didn't manifest themselves in school. When my grandfather gave me a box of old, broken watches, I was fascinated. This was when watches were intricate mysteries of tiny, interacting parts (before the digital revolution). Every time one of his watches broke, if the repair shop could no longer fix it, he would place it in an old cigar box with others facing a similar fate. One day he brought me this "treasure chest" of broken watches. None of the ones in the box ran, and of course they were all too large for me to wear, but that didn't bother me. I wanted to play with them anyway. Which I did. I wound one, and it started to tick. I wound another, and it started, then stopped. A third one wouldn't wind, so I shook it a little. I tightly held the one that started, then stopped, for a few minutes. It started again and continued. I held the one I shook, and it started to work. Soon I was "fixing" my friends' old watches. I guess it's sort of the opposite of whatever principle causes watches to *break* when certain individuals wear them.

But to some people, the ability to repair watches without opening them wasn't as important as the ability to color within the lines and properly recite from *Dick and Jane*. My academic shortcomings were considered severe enough so that when I was in the second or third grade, a social worker came to the house to check out the environment and see why I wasn't achieving in school. Shortly after she arrived, I asked her if she would explain "infinity" to me. Flustered, she jumped to her feet and ran out of the house.

"I'll have to speak to the principal about this," she cried over her shoulder.

If she did so, she never told me what she had learned.

This Time, Closure

There was good reason to contemplate things of an infinite nature, because at this same time, I was about to suffer another loss: my dog. Silk, a Doberman Pinscher, was already two years old at the time I was born, yet she graciously put up with my infantile behavior, including the habit of using her lower lip as a handle with which to pull myself to my feet so I could hold on to her as I was learning to walk. She'd wince with pain, but never would snap or even growl. She somehow knew I was a child and needed her love and protection.

I loved the feel of things that were cool to the touch, including Silk's ears. When she slept next to my bed, I'd drape my arm over the side and gently grip her chilly ear between two fingers. The touching would eventually warm her ear (not what I wanted), so I'd switch to her other ear, then back again when that one got too warm. When both ears had gotten too warm to be interesting, I would let Silk outside to cool off again. After about ten minutes, there'd come a bark at the front door—her signal—and I knew she was ready to come in and do it again. After two complete cycles of this ritual, I would drift off to sleep.

By the time I was 10, Silk was 12 (which is 84 in dog years) and in failing health. My mother and father had made an agreement that, at the point when nothing else could be done for her, they wouldn't let her suffer; they would have her put to sleep.

This had been Silk's most difficult year. There were times when, although she'd try, this dog who helped me learn to walk could simply no longer stand up. It was upsetting for an adult to see this, much less a child. It shook my whole world. It was time to take her to the vet, and we were fairly sure that this was going to be *the* visit.

It was almost Thanksgiving. We decided to wait a day or two until after the holiday. On Thanksgiving day, my mother gave Silk a large platter of turkey with gravy and mashed potatoes and stuffing. Silk, whose diet consisted very little of "people" food, hesitated. Appearing somewhat confused, she looked around at us for approval, then decided not to question it and had her last meal.

The next day, we took her to the vet. My mother stayed home this time. Remembering the lack of closure surrounding the loss of Bubba, I insisted on going along with my father. Sitting in the waiting room with the medicinal smells and the Norman Rockwell–style paintings of dogs playing cards, it all seemed so cold. My father came out and told me that this was it: They were going to put Silk to sleep. Did I want to be there? I followed my father and the vet as they walked Silk through the old hallways and out a back door into a yard. I said good-bye to her, then watched as the vet gave her the needle. After a few seconds, she collapsed gently to the ground. Silk was then lifted up and placed in a cremation unit.

That night and many nights following, I once again cried for a loved one. This time, though, there was closure. Infinity didn't seem so far away, nor eternity so long.

Nature/Nurture

As kindergarten turned into elementary school, my sense of self grew somewhat. I was still bored easily and spent a lot of time daydreaming, but on a rare occasion when I would be assigned a truly inspiring and thought-provoking teacher, I would excel beyond all expectations. Unfortunately, then as today, such teachers were the exception, not the rule.

The atmosphere at home allowed me to develop beyond my years. My parents treated me like an adult: They didn't talk down to me, but included me in conversations and decisions, recognizing me as a person whose opinions mattered.

I couldn't wait to come home from school every day. It seemed that there were always fascinating people to meet. My parents entertained a wide variety of friends with compelling backgrounds: anthropologists, psychologists, artists, doctors, lawyers, and so on. (And to make things even more wonderful, this diverse group inspired an array of delicious cuisine accompanied by delectable tastes and aromas.)

And because my home was so open-minded, and my exposure to people so diverse, it was only natural that I would continue to have a challenge with one-sided, dictatorial authority—or, shall I say, one-sided, dictatorial authority would continue to have a challenge with me.

❧ ❧ ❧

The high school administration was strict about students arriving on time. Although I lived within walking distance of the campus, I was almost always late in the mornings. A minute here, a minute there—no big deal, except to the administration. If students arrived at school after the bell rang, they were expected to get a late pass.

The problem was, the school wouldn't give students a late pass unless they had a note from home. I cut things so closely that I never knew when I was going to be late, and I couldn't get a note from home without walking back there to ask my mother. Accordingly, I would consistently miss the opening half of my first-period class. Why was it so difficult for me to get out of the house just 15 minutes earlier? It didn't make sense—but it didn't change, either. I just didn't seem to operate under the same concept of time as everyone else; I figured that if I left the house every morning at 8:01 A.M. and walked quickly enough, I could arrive at school by 7:50.

Finally, I asked my mother if she'd mind if I wrote my own late notes on those mornings and sign her name on them as necessary. Considering the alternative of my missing an entire subject by walking back and forth every morning, she reluctantly agreed.

One day the school disciplinarian noticed me writing out my own late note. He was a self-styled, ex-military type whose own son could have been the poster child for behavioral problems (makes you think, doesn't it?). Pointing at the note I was writing, he snarled with indignant self-importance, "What are you doing?"

"I'm writing myself a late note," came my calm reply.

"You'll have to come down to the detention room for forging your mother's signature."

"No, I won't. Forgery is without knowledge or consent. And I have both."

Responses like this did not endear me to my teachers. "What's your name?" the disciplinarian demanded.

"Eric Pearl." I stood, gathered my things, and looked the man in the eye. "P-E-A-R-L." Then I turned and walked to my class.

So, between these events—these lessons—my young life went on. My father was part-owner and operator of a vending machine company along with his brother and father. He was also a volunteer policeman. Mom stayed at home and raised the three of us. She also did some part-time modeling and moderated fashion shows. Dad was out of the house by 7:00 A.M., by which time Mom was pushing breakfast down our throats like a mother bird feeding its young. You didn't get out until you ate a good breakfast and had a full lunch box—"all four food groups" (at that time, still a paradigm parents bought into). At age 13, I had my bar-mitzvah. Sometimes on Sundays I attended church with friends.

Kindergarten, elementary school, junior high, high school: new friends, tests, proms, getting my driver's license, SAT's, and finally graduation and college . . .

Moving On

I quickly discovered that graduation from high school didn't mean "freedom"; my parents were determined to keep me close at hand. But as usual, I had different ideas. Why stay in New Jersey? I wanted to go to college in California. You would have thought I'd said "The North Pole."

"It's too far away," my mother and father insisted. Reasonable discussion turned into mounting disagreement, which turned into out-and-out yelling.

In the end, a compromise was reached: I could attend college in Miami, Florida. My parents thought this plan was safe—not only was Miami twice as close to home as California, but my paternal grandfather, Zeida—the one who had given me the box of watches when I was a child—had moved there shortly after Bubba's death. The idea was that Zeida could keep an eye on the prodigal son. I was, after all, the first son of the first son.

This proved to be how my parents lost me for an entire year.

I enrolled at the University of Miami.

My parents had always told me that I could be *anything* I wanted to be, that I could do *anything* I set my mind to do. This was an empowering concept to grow up with, but for me, this lack of an inner compass became more and more of a problem as I grew older and began to think about finding a career. *Be anything* and *do anything* didn't exactly give me much direction. The thing was, nothing interested me, so there was nothing for me to "set my mind to."

I immediately dedicated myself . . . to a completely incoherent course of study. In the space of a year, I considered no fewer than three majors: psychology, pre-law, and modern dance. I had no idea what I wanted to do. And, as always, nothing held my interest for long.

Zeida observed that by living on my own in Miami, I was evolving—and he wanted to see this process continue. Without asking for permission from my parents, he opened the door to the possibility of my spending my sophomore year in the Mediterranean. This was a very exciting prospect. As visions of Rome and Athens floated through my head, Zeida went on to "define" *Mediterranean*. He had a pet name for it. He called it *Israel*. Being one step ahead of the situation, as usual, Zeida produced a brochure for a one-year course of study in Jerusalem, a program for American students. He then offered to subsidize the venture. How could my parents say no?

More Than Milk and Honey

Most of the students traveling to Israel went there expecting God to descend from the heavens, and for milk and honey to flow in the streets. They were disappointed. However, I went there expecting little more than a year outside of the U.S., so without unrealistic expectations to get in my way, I ended up falling in love with *everything*. Up until then, that trip to the Holy Land was the most powerful year of my life. To this day, I awaken from dreams where I'm still there among the people, the ancient temples, and the breathtaking views from Mt. Sinai.

Upon my return to the States, I stepped back into the exact same life I had left behind. Whatever I had found in the Holy Land hadn't revealed my true purpose—or if it had, I didn't recognize it. Now I was back to facing my dilemma: selecting a major.

An idea had occurred to me the year before leaving on my trip. During my year in Miami, I'd had an experience with Rolfing, a type of deep-tissue massage designed to free up the musculature of the body. Some friends of mine had gone through the ten prescribed Rolfing sessions, and I had seen the physical changes it brought about in them. Their before-and-after pictures were all I needed to decide to get "Rolfed," also.

The sessions ended up changing the way I held myself and seemed to open me up to a more expansive way of viewing the world. Built on the concept of a mind/body feedback loop, the theory behind Rolfing is that it frees up your individual muscles, and in the process, releases stored pain— physical and emotional, old and new. Oftentimes, as you go through these sessions, you relive past experiences as their discomfort leaves you. As a result, both your physical body and emotions are often transformed. This new existence, free from many of your older pains, allows you to move, stand, and hold yourself differently. And when you hold yourself differently—that is, when you occupy a different physical space—you occupy a different emotional space as well.

Impressed by both the concept and the results, I thought about becoming a Rolfer myself. But my parents felt that Rolfing might turn out to be a fad, fall out of fashion, and leave me professionally stranded. Perhaps, they suggested, I should consider entering a health-care field that was more proven: chiropractic. If nothing else, at least I'd have a degree to fall back upon.

I agreed to travel to Brooklyn and speak to a chiropractor I was introduced to by a friend of the family. The doctor related the basic philosophy behind the art and science of chiropractic. He explained that there is a universal intelligence that maintains the organization and balance of the universe; and that there's an extension of that intelligence, called *innate intelligence*, within each of us, keeping us alive, healthy, and in balance. This innate intelligence, or life force, communicates with the rest of our physical being in large part via our brain, spinal cord, and the rest of our nervous system—the controlling system of our body. As long as the communication between our brain and our body is open and flowing freely, we remain in our optimum potential state of health.

When one of the vertebrae twists or moves out of position, it can result in pressure on our nerves, inhibiting or cutting off communication between the part of us supplied by those specific nerves, and our brain. As a result of this interference, our cells may begin to break down and our resistance may weaken, allowing for *dis*-ease, the predecessor of disease. What a chiropractor does, then, is remove the interference caused by these misalignments (called *subluxations*) in our spine, and allow our life force to take over once again, bringing us back into a healthy state of balance. In other words, this is healing by way of removing the cause, not covering up or treating the symptom.

When I suddenly realized that people's headaches weren't the result of congenital blood-aspirin deficiencies—as our television commercials would lead us to believe—and that there was something that I could do to help, I made up my mind to become a chiropractor. I didn't stop to contemplate the enormity of this step, nor did I foresee the role it would ultimately play in my life. Synchronicity wasn't a concept consciously entertained.

All of a sudden, something "clicked." I was flooded with childhood memories of fantasies—or were they visions?—of helping people as the Oracle of Delphi. Maybe this was a way for me to actually do something along those lines. All I knew at that moment was that something in what the doctor had said struck a chord. Something about this felt perfect—and that was enough for me. I was about to take my first step in a new direction—one that would ultimately bring me closer to my destiny.

❦ ❦ ❦

CHAPTER FOUR

A New Path of Discovery

"Of course you're psychic; you just don't realize it."
— my friend Debbie Luican

Back to School

The Brooklyn chiropractor I'd spoken with had recommended Cleveland Chiropractic College in Los Angeles. I applied there and was accepted.

And so it happened that my parents lost a son after all—and lost him to California, where he'd wanted to go all along. On the other hand, they eventually gained a doctor, so I guess it all balanced out.

I'll always remember my first day at chiropractic college. The freshman class was large, more than 80 students. A temporary wall had to be opened so we could spill into a second room. The instructor asked each of us to briefly state his or her reason for wanting to be a chiropractor. He began with the student sitting at the far left end of the first row, who, of course, happened to be farthest from where I sat, in the rear right-hand corner of the room. From there, the storytelling crisscrossed the rows of students. I sat and listened to story after story of how this student was paralyzed until a visit to a chiropractor; that student's cancer disappeared; this one had her vision restored; that other one was relieved of lifelong migraines—on and on, a never-ending litany of permanent healings beyond the realm of what any non-chiropractor was used to hearing. Especially me. Zeida still called chiropractors "back-crackers."

Finally, it was my turn to speak. Eighty-three heads turned to hear my story—the last one of the day. Was mine really going to be the climactic epic that would launch the other students out of the room and onto their shining new paths in life? I think not. I was the only person in the class who had never even visited a chiropractor. For that matter, I still didn't really know what a chiropractor was. I just remembered bits and pieces of what that doctor had told me during our 20 minutes together—something about removing the interference and allowing the body to heal itself. The premise made such perfect sense when it was explained to me that I never bothered to test it out, to look into it, or to talk to others about it. I rose, looked across the crowd, and heard myself say, "Well . . . it *sounded* good."

If You Can't Find It, You're Trying Too Hard

So here I was, back in school—but things were a little different this time. For once, this was a school and a course of study *I'd* chosen. That made a world of difference.

Not being a bookworm, I enjoyed socializing, partying, and exploring my new city. I took a part-time job in a shoe store because, although my parents sent me money to cover my educational expenses, I wanted to earn a few extra dollars to do the things that *I* wanted to do. One day, a customer—a researcher from a seismology lab—came in to buy shoes. In the course of shopping, he happened to mention that, at the lab, they were anticipating an earthquake for the southern California area within the next 24 hours.

"Did you tell any of the other employees?" I asked.

"No, I didn't."

"Good. Don't." I smiled. He smiled back, understanding, then paid for his shoes and left.

A few minutes after he left the store, I pretended to have a premonition and announced to my co-workers that I had a *feeling* there was going to be an earthquake in three days.

As "predicted," it happened. Everyone felt it, and it was on the news. My co-workers were very impressed.

A few days later, and without the intervention of a seismologist, I got the feeling that there was going to be another quake. Bravely, I took a chance and announced this one, too.

Believe it or not, we had another one.

It was as if something had been triggered inside me. During the next two or three years, I accurately predicted 21 out of 24 earthquakes.

One afternoon, my roommate came home to find a note I'd left him: *The earth is going to shake*. He told me later that the quake had struck at the same moment he was reading the note. His girlfriend was standing next to him the entire time . . . screaming.

On another day, as I was eating alone in a restaurant, I felt the beginnings of another earthquake, the kind that makes a "rolling" movement. As its intensity increased, I looked around the room. No one else was reacting. No one's water glass was shaking; the lamps hung motionless overhead. Yet at the same time, *I* could see the lamps swinging. It was real for *me*. I got up and hurried out onto the street. I couldn't figure out why no one else was fleeing, why on all sides of me life was going on with the monotonous normalcy of Mayberry.

It seemed impossible. The earth was still shaking; I could *feel* it. It was the longest rolling earthquake I'd ever been in; yet the combination of its surreal movement and the fact that no one else seemed to notice it made me conclude that it must not be happening after all. I sheepishly returned to the restaurant. I was glad I'd been dining alone; explaining my abrupt flight into the street might have been a bit . . . difficult.

But if that hadn't been a real quake, then it must have been another premonition. There was no other explanation.

On the way home from the restaurant, I stopped at the cleaners to pick up my laundry and mentioned to the owners that the earth was going to shake that night. They all laughed.

Later that evening, the quake hit. Its epicenter was in Culver City, right where the people who owned the cleaners lived.

A few weeks later, after I'd stored up enough dirty laundry to fill a half-dozen king-sized pillowcases, I went back to the cleaners. Struggling to peer above the first set of three that I carried in my arms, I felt for the door with my foot. Carefully nudging it open, I was engrossed in the process of trying to locate the counter with my toes. Suddenly, a voice rang out so loudly I'm surprised I didn't throw all three bags of laundry into the air.

"That's him! That's the one!" shouted the woman behind the counter in a heavy Russian-Jewish accent. "Here's my address," she said as she shoved a hastily scribbled piece of paper into my hand. "I vant you should give me a phone call before the next one comes!"

From then on, anytime I entered that store, I was asked to predict the next quake. And I would try, too—but it didn't seem to work out that way. I couldn't force it; the predictions only came when I was minding my own business.

Without realizing it, I'd learned a profound truth: *If you can't find it, you're trying too hard.*

Resurrection

Now and then I'd scrape together enough money from my student budget to attend a double feature at the theater around the corner from my apartment. One afternoon I arrived just in time for the second feature, or "B," film—*Resurrection*, starring Ellen Burstyn. Of course, it was a "B" movie in placement only, because Ms. Burstyn would go on to be nominated for an Academy Award for best actress for her role in the film.

Resurrection is based on the story of a woman named Edna Mae, who, after an automobile accident, dies in the operating room . . . only to come back to life. Sometime later, she discovers that she has the power of healing—a sort-of "laying-on of hands." Just by touching people and simultaneously entering into a state of love, they would have healings. Sometimes she would take on their illness or infirmity—having removed it from the other person—and then release the symptoms from her own body. Other times, the healings would seem to occur as if by grace, without her having to take anything on.

I was so fascinated by this film that after sitting through the first feature—whatever it was—I watched *Resurrection* again. Then I brought my friends to see it. Later I brought more friends. I had no idea why I was so compelled to see this film over and over again. At the time, although the healing aspect of the movie was interesting, what really got me was the similarity between the film's portrayal of Edna Mae's near-death experience, and what my mother had gone through the day I was born. I had never seen or read anything on this subject, and this film so accurately described my mom's experience. Every time I watched it, I felt as if I were getting a glimpse into something that was somehow very familiar. It was as if I could almost see something, almost remember something. Something . . .

Other Hints

During my time of exploration, I also discovered what's called "psychometry," the ability or art of gathering information about people by touching or holding an object belonging to them, usually a piece of jewelry that they've worn. After seeing someone do this, I tried it myself and found that it opened me up to receive some remarkably accurate insights into people, some of whom I'd never met. During my brief foray into this process, I discovered two "secrets" about it: The more consistently I kept my fingers moving on the piece of jewelry, the more focused I would become; and the faster I spoke, the more accurate the information. The persistent exploration of the object with my fingers seemed to still my mind, in a similar fashion to the way, for many of us, our minds become relaxed and quieted when we drive. The quicker speech apparently didn't allow me time to second-guess myself. Through the stillness of my mind came the insights; through the quickness of my speech came the courage to voice them.

I mention these points not just because they were strange to me, but because they hinted at "other" influences in my life, even in those early years.

Aside from these somewhat colorful events, my main activity during this period of time was the very thing my primary and secondary school teachers would never have believed: I attended classes and studied. Well, okay, my version of "attending class" often consisted of my sitting in the back of the room and raising my arm just long enough to say, "Here." Still, as in my earlier school career, I managed to get good grades . . . and I finally graduated with a degree in chiropractic.

I'd unintentionally proven my childhood school director right. I'd found something that interested me, and I was going to make something of my life after all.

Fevers and Visitors

One day in 1983, not long after I graduated from college, I realized that I was feeling a little under the weather: achy, headachy, and feverish. I wasn't a big fan of taking aspirin to bring down a fever, as I knew that fevers had their purpose and I wanted to allow this one to run its course. Accordingly, I got into bed, bundled up, drank plenty of fluids—and watched TV (guilt-free television: the definite high point of being home in bed, sick). But after a few days, I decided that it was time to do something more active to break the fever. So every night I'd pile on the comforter and blankets, sweat it out, and change sheets and pajamas at least twice.

Every morning I'd wake up no better than the day before. Finally, I gave in and called a medical doctor. He prescribed Tylenol with codeine. These must have been the number-four Tylenol-with-codeines—the *really big* ones—because it takes a heck of a lot of codeine to knock me out during an *I Love Lucy* marathon. But let me tell you, after I popped those pills, the entire day was a blur of red hair and Cuban accents.

My temperature was way up there: 105, 106, 107. Finally, after yet another night of changing sheets and pajamas (I was sure that if I just continued the pattern, the fever would break), I opened my eyes, and for the briefest moment, saw that I had "company." There, at the foot of my bed, stood a group of "people." There appeared to be about seven of them, varying in size and shape: some tall, some short, and one almost dwarflike. They remained there just long enough for me to see them, and for them to *see* that I saw them.

Then they were gone.

Before my mind could consciously process what had just occurred, I drew in a breath. That breath felt analogous to a newborn's first inhalation in that it seemed as if it was my very first breath of the day—as though, from the time I opened my eyes until the time my "visitors" left, I hadn't breathed. As I began to inhale, I felt—and heard—a tiny rattling sound in my chest. Suddenly I understood: *I'm dying.*

I called my M.D. and told him I was coming right over, then phoned a taxi service and requested that they send a car with air-conditioning because we were in a summer heat wave, and with my fever, I was in a heat wave of my own.

I could hardly stand, but I made it to the door and out to the street. The cab arrived . . . no air-conditioning, of course. Delirious, I climbed in anyway.

At his office, my doctor x-rayed my lungs and told me to go directly to the hospital. "Do not stop along the way," he said. It appeared that I had pneumonia. Sensing that more than a brief visit awaited me, I nonetheless took a cab straight home so that I could collect my pajamas, toothbrush, and so on.

I had no health insurance at the time, so I was kept waiting for quite a while at the county hospital before being admitted into the ward. The next morning, they moved me into a room where I stayed for ten days of tubes, oxygen . . . and food worthy of a domestic airline. When I was finally released, my weight had dropped to 138 pounds—and I'm six feet tall. My M.D. later confessed that he thought I might not make it out of there alive.

I don't remember much about my time in the hospital, but I do know I lost a good deal of my short-term memory, probably as a result of running such a high-grade fever.

(Speaking of overheated brains, have you ever noticed how similar the words *perspiration* and *apparition* are to one another? They both have two *I*'s, two *P*'s, five vowels, four syllables . . . and either one can bring about the other.) So who *were* those people I saw standing at the foot of my bed at home? Were they guides? Spirits? Guardian angels? Were they an inter-dimensional group of observers? Were they apparitions caused by my fever—in other words, a delusion? Or, were they apparitions that truly existed but which only my fever allowed me to see—that is, beings who dwelled on a plane within one of those 11 (so far) theorized planes of exis-tence (according to today's tenets of quantum thought)?

I don't know. But one thing's for sure: If I hadn't seen those visitors on the day my chest rattled, I would have just continued my regimen of drinking juice and bundling up—and I most certainly would have died.

That wasn't something I was ready to do, though. I had other plans. And maybe, just maybe, someone or something had plans for me, too.

Resurrection—Again

As part of the professional process I'd selected, I finally became an "extern"; in effect, a "student doctor" at a licensed chiropractor's office. Although rewarding in many ways, this phase of a new chiropractor's career was not exactly what you'd call lucrative. Like most people, I assumed all doctors knew how to run an office. I was wrong. In the practice I joined, there were a lot of things they didn't know. Patient relations was at the top of the list. Our agreement was that I paid them 50 percent of what I col-lected from my patients. Since they treated their own patients, shall we say, less than royally, it was no surprise then, that they treated mine only half as well. And, because of the way they treated my patients, a lot of them never came back.

With an income of only 50 percent of what I was taking in and an unpre-dictable patient base, I could barely pay the rent at either the office or my apartment. The longer I worked as an extern, the more money I owed. The more money I owed, the less I could afford to leave—until after three years, I *had* to leave—or give up my career entirely.

So I left.

I did, however, reap a couple of fringe benefits from that experience. One of my patients happened to be pivotally connected to the movie *Res-urrection,* which, as I mentioned, had become one of my favorites. Another patient happened to be a member of the Academy of Motion Picture Arts and Sciences, and she took me to the Academy Awards that year. So there I was, sitting in the balcony watching the proceedings. As I turned around, I saw that Ellen Burstyn, a nominee who had been seated up front on the main floor, had come up and taken the seat just behind me. *How strange*, I thought. I hadn't noticed that seat open earlier in the evening.

After a while, she got up and left. I never again saw her in person, nor did I think much about that near-encounter, or the other odd events that had marked my life: the "beings" at the foot of my bed, the earthquake predictions, the psychometry, the watches "fixing" themselves. . . .

At least I didn't think much about them until 13 years later, when the healings began.

The Ghost of Melrose Place

As an ex-extern, without much time or money, I grabbed the first location that fit my budget—one bedroom in a converted two-bedroom upstairs apartment on Melrose Place that I shared with two psychologists. Melrose Place—all three blocks of it—was considered by many to be one of the most interesting and upscale streets in Los Angeles, but obviously, the people who made these assessments had never seen my new office. Making patients schlep up a flight of stairs wasn't the only problem with it. As everyone knows, nobody goes anywhere in L.A. except by car, and parking on Melrose Place was almost nonexistent—which inspired me to make parking arrangements with some of the people who owned the fine antique and art stores along the block. And that's how it came to be that my more social-climbing patients could boast that their chiropractor had valet parking.

But all that came later. In the beginning, my greatest problem was figuring out how to transform a single bedroom into useful chiropractic space. Designing a series of oddly shaped treatment cubicles, I created three rooms out of the bedroom, turned the "breakfast room" into a reception area, and crammed a desk and a receptionist into the tiniest kitchen space you can imagine. Then I hired contractors to do the work.

As anyone who's ever dealt with construction knows, the work can just run on and on, going way over budget and over schedule. Eventually I ran out of money, and I couldn't talk the bank into loaning me more.

Every morning I came to my half-finished office to see patients and do two other things: call the bank to try to talk them into lending me more money, and tighten the screws in my new track lighting. At $27 for one track light and four 'cans, the idea of recessed lighting had gone right out the window along with the contractor's estimated fees and their completion dates.

For some reason, every single morning those track-light screws came "unscrewed" and extended a good three-quarters of an inch from their fully tightened positions. I was on the corner of a heavily trafficked street; therefore, the traffic vibrations might have been what was loosening them. Just the same, every morning I would retighten the screws. It was a cycle: The bank tightened the screws on me, and I tightened the screws on my track lighting.

Late one night, after my "staff" (a woman who spent so much time filing her nails I was surprised there wasn't blood on everything she touched) had locked up and gone home, I remained to adjust a late-arriving patient. Movement caught my eye, and I looked up as a man strolled down the hall past the doorway of the adjusting room. I knew that the main door to the suite was locked, so there was no way anyone could have gotten in. Yet I saw this man quite clearly: He stood about 5'10", with a round face and close-cropped, wavy hair. He wore a gray textured overcoat, and looked to be in his late 20s or early 30s.

I knew without a doubt that he was a ghost.

The next morning when I told the psychologists who shared the apartment about this, I was amazed to find that they were both already aware of this visitor. They hadn't mentioned him to me because they needed a third person to share the rent and were afraid that the prospect of a ghost would scare me off.

The truth was, I didn't really mind the ghost—but he seemed to mind me. "Too much foot traffic," said one medium who felt he could get the ghost to leave. "He doesn't mind one-person-per-hour for the psychologists, but you're bringing too many strangers into his home."

I watched as this person walked through the apartment (my office), found the spot where he felt the ghost spent most of his time, and very politely informed the ghost that it was dead. After that, he told it to "Go into the light," or something like that. It took all of about 30 seconds.

That was on a Sunday night. The next morning, I walked in and noticed my light fixtures: They were all screwed in nice and tight, and stayed that way until I took them down five years later as part of an office expansion.

Then the phone rang. It was my bank. My loan had come through.

\mathfrak{Se} CHAPTER FIVE \mathfrak{Se}

Opening New Doors,
Turning on the Light

"What lies behind us and what lies before
us are tiny matters compared to what lies within us."
— Ralph Waldo Emerson

The Jewish Gypsy of Venice Beach

Twelve years passed, and by then I'd taken over about half of the second floor of the Melrose Place building for my practice. Things were booming. The office featured eight adjustment rooms and was kept lively with assistants, massage therapists, foot reflexologists, parking valets, and as many patients as I could handle. Yet, emotionally, I was barely holding on.

I had just ended a six-year relationship that I'd fully expected to last the rest of my life. Somehow I stumbled through the days after the breakup, virtually unable to place one foot in front of the other. The only thing more difficult than waking up every morning to go into the office was keeping it together for the patients while I was there.

As if there wasn't enough going on in my personal life, it so happened that at this very same time, I was in the process of hiring a completely new staff. An exceedingly competent woman who had been managing my office moved to a different part of the state to be with her boyfriend. The timing of this move coincided with another mutually agreed-upon departure or two. Soon I was starting fresh. It took two people to replace the manager who left—one to handle the behind-the-scenes things such as insurance billing, medical reports, and correspondence; the other to handle patient relations and office flow. This position was called *front desk*.

\mathfrak{Se} 43 \mathfrak{Se}

Like a Broadway show (or, in this case, a soap opera), the work had to go on, so I started interviewing people for the front-desk position. I had always liked "personality" in a receptionist, as a *sociable* personality at the front desk creates a bond with the patients, and a *strong* personality keeps me from getting bored.

I had never done a particularly great job of hiring people, so a friend of mine who did that kind of thing professionally came in to help me interview. One or two other people also assisted in the screening process. As we went through the applicants, one woman stood out in my mind—and everyone else's. Believe it or not, she looked, sounded, and *behaved* like Fran Drescher's character in the TV show *The Nanny*: Tall, dark-haired, and attractive, she had a flip attitude; a high-pitched, nasal, New York accent; and a voice that could shatter diamonds. She was a no-longer-aspiring actress (if there is such a thing).

Everyone said, "Don't hire her. Don't hire that woman." But I had to have her. For one thing, something about her eyes reminded me of Bubba. For another, I couldn't believe that such a person could truly exist. I tried one last time to talk myself out of hiring her, to listen to the voices of experience who had come to help me select competent office staff, but I was fascinated by her. There was no use clouding the issue with logic.

It turned into a true love/hate relationship. I loved her. The patients hated her.

One day she announced that, with all the stress I'd been under, a day at the beach would do me good. What that really meant was that *she* wanted to go to the beach and didn't want to spend her own money on gasoline, but what the heck. That Saturday, off we went to Venice Beach. We spent some time just relaxing on the sand, then she wandered off. When she came back, she said, "There's this woman reading cards. You need to get your cards read by her."

I didn't have anything against having my cards read, but I really preferred to go to someone who came with a better recommendation.

"I don't want to get my cards read by some character on the beach," I responded.

If a reader were all that wonderful, people would come to see her, I thought to myself. *She wouldn't be dragging a card table, tablecloth, chairs, and other accoutrements to an overcrowded beach sidewalk in an attempt to flag people down for readings.*

But my receptionist pushed and pushed in that very "Nanny" fashion. One look into her eyes told me that further protest would prove fruitless.

Eventually she confessed that she had met this woman at a party and told her that we'd be at the beach this day. "I'd be very embarrassed if you didn't get a reading," she whined, wrinkling her brow. *"Pulllease . . ."*

Surrendering, I followed "Nanny" across the hot sand of the beach to see this woman. There she sat behind a card table with her cards spread out in an appropriately gypsylike manner. After being introduced, she said, "Bubbelah, we've got $10 readings and $20 readings."

Bubbelah? Was there really such a thing as a Jewish gypsy?

I had somehow come to the beach with only $20 in my pocket. Thinking about how hungry I was, I said, "I'll take the $10 reading."

In exchange for my money, I received a very nice yet not really memorable, present-time reading. When it was over, almost as an afterthought, the woman said, "There's very special work that I do. It reconnects your body's meridian lines to the grid lines on the planet, which connects us to the stars and other planets." She told me that as a healer, it was something that I needed. She also told me I could read about it in a work called *The Book of Knowledge: The Keys of Enoch,* by J. J. Hurtak. It sounded quite interesting, so I asked *the* question: "How much?" She said, "$333." I said, "No, thank you."

This is the kind of stuff you're warned about on the evening news. I can hear the blurb now: "Jewish gypsy on Venice Beach takes $333 from unsuspecting chiropractor . . ." My picture with the word *Sucker* under it flashes across the screen. ". . . convinces doctor to pay her an additional $150 a month for life to burn candles for his protection . . . film at 11:00." I felt humiliated for even having considered it. So, my receptionist and I left and creatively went about constructing a $10 lunch for two.

You'd think this would be the end of it, but the mind works in mysterious ways. I couldn't get the woman's words out of my head. I found myself taking the last few minutes of a lunch break to go to the Bodhi Tree bookstore near my office, attempting to quickly read through Chapter 3.1.7 of *The Book of Knowledge: The Keys of Enoch.* (This was the chapter recommended to me that day on the beach.) The greatest lesson that day, however, was that if ever a book was created that could not be quickly read through, this was the one. But I'd read enough. This was going to haunt me until I gave in. I cracked open my cookie jar and gave the woman a call.

The work was to be done over two days, two days apart. On day one, I gave her my money, lay there on her table, and listened to my mind jabber while she dimmed the lights and put on the New Age tinkle music. *This is the dumbest thing I've ever done,* I thought to myself. *I can't believe I paid this kind of money to a perfect stranger so she could draw lines on my body with her fingertips.* As I lay there thinking of all the good uses this money could've been put toward, a sudden surge of insight came over me, and I heard myself think, *Well, you've already given her the money. You may as well cut the negative chatter and be open to receiving whatever there is to receive.* So I lay there quietly, ready and open. When it was over, my mind announced that I had experienced nothing. *Absolutely nothing.* I, however, was the only one in the room who seemed to know this. The woman sat me up as if the earth had moved, telling me to hold on to her as she proceeded to slowly walk me around her living room.

"Ground yourself," she instructed me. "Come back into your body."

And then I heard it: that not-so-quiet little voice inside my head saying, *Lady, I don't know what you think went on here, but I missed it.*

I had paid for both sessions, so I decided I might as well come back on Sunday for part two. The strangest thing happened that night, however. About an hour after I'd gone to sleep, the lamp next to my bed—one I'd had for ten years—turned itself on, and I woke up to the very real sensation that there were people in my home. So I got up bravely—with a carving knife, a can of pepper spray, and my Doberman Pinscher—and searched the house. But I found no one. I went back to bed with the uncanniest feeling that I wasn't alone, that I was being watched.

✐ ✐ ✐

My next session started out pretty much the same as the first. However, it soon became apparent that it was to be anything but. My legs didn't want to stay still. They had that "crazy leg" feeling that strikes some people every once in a blue moon in the middle of the night. Soon that sensation took over the rest of my body, interspersed with almost unbearable chills. It was all I could do to lie still on the table. Much as I wanted to jump up and down and shake the feeling out of every cell in my body, I didn't dare move. Why? Because I had given the woman more money than I spend on a week's worth of groceries, and I intended to get every penny's worth out of the experience—*that's why.*

The session finally ended. It was an oppressively hot August day, and we were in a non-air-conditioned apartment. Yet I was chilled near frozen, my teeth chattering as this woman rushed to wrap me in a blanket, where I remained for a good five minutes until my body temperature returned to normal.

I was now different. I don't understand what happened, nor could I possibly attempt to explain it, yet I was no longer the person I was four days prior. I somehow made it to my car, which seemed to know the way home on its own.

I don't remember anything about the rest of that day. I couldn't tell you for certain if the rest of the day even took place. All I do know is that the following morning I found myself at work.

My odyssey had begun.

Something Was Up

My memory returned at the point where I stepped into the reception area of my office. It was as if a part of my brain had been lifted out of my skull the previous day and had just now been returned to me.

But that wasn't the only strange thing. I also found myself fielding a barrage of unanticipated questions: "What happened to you over the weekend? You look so different! You *sound* so different!" I certainly wasn't going to respond by saying, *"Oh, I paid a fortuneteller at the beach $333 to draw lines on my body with her fingertips; why do you ask?"*

Some questions are best left unanswered.

"Oh, nothing," I casually replied, wondering myself exactly what had taken place over the weekend.

It had been my practice to have my patients lie on the table with their eyes closed for 30 to 60 seconds following their adjustments. This allowed them time to relax while their adjustments "set." On this particular Monday, seven of my patients—some of whom had been with me for more than a decade, and one who was seeing me for the first time—asked me if I had been walking around the table as they lay there. Some asked if anyone else had come into the room, because it felt as if several people were standing or walking around the table. Three said it felt as if people were *running* around the table, and two sheepishly confided that it seemed as if people were *flying* around the table.

I'd been a chiropractor for 12 years, and no one had ever expressed anything like this before. Now, seven people had said this to me on the same day. It didn't take a piano to fall on my head. *Something was up!*

My patients were reporting that they could tell where my hands were before I touched their body. They could feel my hands when they were inches to feet away from them. It became a game to see how accurately they could locate my hands. Yet it became *more* than a game as people started receiving healings. At first, the healings were less dramatic: aches, pains, and the like. As patients would come in for chiropractic, I would adjust them, then tell them to close their eyes and lie there until I told them to open them again. While their eyes were closed, I would pass my hands over the patients for a moment or two. When they got up and realized that their pain was gone, they asked me what I had done.

"Nothing—and don't tell anyone!" became my standard reply. This directive was about as effective as Nancy Reagan's "Just Say No" approach to drugs.

Soon, patients were coming in from all over for these "healings." I had very little idea what was going on with all of this, as no one had seen fit to leave me a book of instructions. Sure, I checked in regularly with the woman in Venice Beach—I had to talk to *someone,* because strange things were going on in my house, too, and I couldn't really mention these phenomena to any of my "sane" friends.

"It must have come from something that was already in you," she told me. Then she added, "Maybe it has something to do with your mother's near-death experience at the time of your birth. This is so unusual. Nothing like this has ever happened before."

That first day on the beach, she had suggested I start taking "flower essence drops" and had intuited the specific drops she wanted me to take. Actually, she had intuited six, but told me that I was only to blend five of them at a time.

So I went through the process of determining which five to take and which one to leave out. This decision-making procedure could be either very funny—or very annoying to anyone who knew me at that time because . . . well . . . let's just say I wasn't known for my decisiveness.

I finally sent away for my drops, and when they arrived, I mixed them in my kitchen with a degree of care bordering on reverence. I filled a one-ounce dropper bottle three-quarters full of spring water. I added seven drops of each of the five flower essences I'd decided upon into each of the little bottles. I kept one bottle by my bed, one in my briefcase, one in my medicine cabinet, and one in the desk drawer at my office. In near-sacramental fashion, I placed seven drops of my newly made concoction under my tongue four times each day, and if that weren't enough, I took a bath (clear water, the juice of half a lemon, and seven drops of the medley) every three days. For 20 minutes, I would soak in the tub, carefully rewetting all the parts of my head and body that might begin to air-dry, such as my nose (which

I later realized had to stay above water a large part of the time). The woman's instructions were precise, and I followed them maybe even more precisely than was necessary.

Why do I mention this? Because it seemed that on these ritual nights, after I had gone through my usual routine of locking and relocking, alarm setting and resetting, and finally going to sleep, I would awaken to the experience of people being in my home. I would get up, heart pounding, and go through the house, feeling that at any minute I would come upon someone who wasn't there when I went to sleep . . . only to discover that a door that I had closed was now open and/or a light that I had turned off prior to going to bed was now on.

Doors opening and lights coming on—nice metaphor. Yet I wasn't looking at it from a sufficient distance to recognize it as such. I just knew that something out of the ordinary was occurring in my home and I wanted answers. My gypsy didn't have them for me, but she didn't seem worried about what was happening, so neither was I.

Little did I know that soon we were about to pass out of her area of familiarity altogether.

Blisters and Bleeding

Some patients still came in for standard chiropractic treatment, unaware of the "other things" that were going on in my office. One of these patients had been referred to me by her orthopedist, who hadn't been able to resolve her back pain. The woman was in her late 40s and had suffered from this pain for a long time. It was particularly bad the day she arrived, but not just in her back. She told me she'd had a degenerative bone disease of her right knee since she was nine years old, and that the pain in her knee was almost intolerable.

I adjusted her, then told her to close her eyes and not open them until I asked her to. While her eyes were shut, I walked around to her right knee and held my hands maybe six inches above it, moving them in small circles. I'd noticed that there was always some kind of sensation in my hands when I did this with a person, and this time the feeling was heat. That's all I noticed: heat—although maybe just a bit more heat than usual.

After I finished, I asked her to open her eyes. When she did, she told me she felt better. I must admit, I was getting sort of used to this type of response by now. Strange as it was, it seemed to be happening with a great deal of regularity. It's what happened next that really surprised me. We walked toward the front door, and as we approached the front desk, my receptionist nearly fell out of her chair.

"Look!" she squealed in her unique fashion as she pointed at my hand. I looked down. My palm was covered with blisters—tiny, millimeter-sized blisters. Seventy-five, one-hundred, maybe more. Within three to four hours, they were gone.

This blistering occurred on more than one occasion. And in a way, I welcomed it—it was a visible manifestation of something otherwise unseen. This was something I could show people and say, "See? See?"

Then it happened. My palm bled. I kid you not. Instead of blistering, it bled. Not streams outpouring, as in old movies or the *National Enquirer,* but more as if I'd stuck my palm with a pin. Yet it was blood just the same.

As my patient and I both stared silently at it, some other patients crept closer.

"It's an initiation," one of them said.

"Into what?" I asked.

No one could say.

And, again, how would *they* know? Why didn't *I* know? Who *really* knows?

Looking for Answers

My quest for explanations not only continued, it accelerated. I discovered the names and backgrounds of some of the people renowned for their expertise in various areas of spiritual and so-called paranormal phenomena. I'd buy their audio books and listen to them in my car; and I'd come up with questions I wanted to ask them.

And now and then, I'd succeed in doing so.

When I heard that Brian Weiss, M.D., author of *Many Lives, Many Masters,* would be teaching a one-day seminar, I immediately made arrangements to attend. Dr. Weiss is one of the world's foremost authorities on past-life regression. He started his career as a conventional psychiatrist and hypnotherapist, but in the course of treating certain patients, he became convinced of the reality of past lives and the effect they can have on one's present one.

I hoped that if I attended his seminar, I'd be able to speak with him during a break to see if he could shed some light on what was happening in my own once-normal life.

Well, there was a break all right, but not the kind I anticipated.

I sat through the day's seminar with approximately 600 other people, all of whom were hungrily waiting to speak to Dr. Weiss personally in the hopes that he would not only be riveted by what they had to say, but would take the time to speak with them so that they could feel important. Apparently, few realized—or cared—that 600 people asking questions multiplied by one minute per answer equals ten hours, which would have been longer than the time allotted for the entire seminar.

Of course, I was one of those people. And like the rest, I felt that my question *had* to be asked. So I waited for appropriate hand-raising opportunities: natural breaks in the flow of the lecture, topics related to my question, et cetera. The second option should have offered many jumping-in places, because I'd have to preface my question with a brief history of what had been going on with me—events that touched on almost every topic Dr. Weiss had been discussing.

Yet questions were not only *not* being taken, they weren't even invited.

Soon came the midday break. The seminar was half over, and I still hadn't successfully created my opportunity.

After the break, Dr. Weiss announced that he was going to do a past-life regression on stage and needed a volunteer from the audience. Five hundred and ninety-seven hands went up (three people must have still been in the bathroom). Dr. Weiss announced that he would select five people from the audience to come up, then perform some sort of eye test on each of them to determine who would be his best subject. The other four would be returned to their seats.

"One, two, three, four, five . . ." Dr. Weiss hand-picked his volunteers and up they came, each taking one of the five designated positions. None of them was me.

Those of us not selected lowered our hands and anxiously waited to see what would happen next . . . when suddenly Dr. Weiss turned back toward the audience, scanning it as if he had lost something. "You!" He pointed through the crowd. "Didn't you have your hand up?"

As I looked around to see whom he was pointing at, I realized that everyone else was staring at *me*.

"Yes," I blurted, embarrassed and not quite knowing what to do with myself. "But you already picked five people."

"Did you want to come up?"

Of course I wanted to come up. What kind of a question was that?

"Well, yes," I replied.

"Okay, then come up," he told me.

To say that I now wanted to crawl into a hole would give a whole new level of meaning to the word *understatement*. Somehow it seemed a lot easier to think of being one of a group of five than a lone individual being so blatantly singled out.

But I went—after receiving a few friendly elbows in the ribs and a couple of not-so-well-disguised dirty looks. I couldn't blame them. Everyone wanted to be regressed by Brian Weiss.

Dr. Weiss brought me up and described the "eye test" he was going to conduct on each of us. It was basically a susceptibility-to-hypnosis test where we looked way up without moving our heads, then slowly closed our eyes so he could see the "flutter." From this he could evidently determine who would be the most susceptible to hypnotic regression.

If you haven't already guessed, I was the lucky one. Maybe he knew it all along.

He sat me on a stool, had me close my eyes, made a few suggestions, then asked, "What is it that you see?"

I realized that I was looking down at myself, even though my eyes were closed. I saw tanned skin, but of a different tone than mine—it was an olive, Mediterranean complexion. Suddenly I knew that I was a young boy living in some distant era somewhere in the desert. I also knew that by today's standards, I looked older than I actually was. In fact, according to what I said out loud to Dr. Weiss and the audience, I was "a young boy between the ages of 12 and 17."

I described my surroundings: the interior courtyard of a very large building featuring stone columns. One column stood in the middle of the courtyard, rising higher than my eyes could see. It was enormous, five feet in diameter, big enough for me to hide behind, which was what I was doing. At this point, my mouth told the audience, "I'm back in Egypt," while in my mind, I was thinking, *God! Egypt! Everyone says they go back to Egypt. Am I making this up?* I continued by saying, "I'm living in the house of the Pharaoh." *Of course I am. How unimaginative of me.* "I'm immediate family of the Pharaoh." *So now I'm royalty.* "Yet I'm not blood of the Pharaoh." *And now I suppose I'm Moses. I can't believe I'm saying this.*

There was a story unfolding in my mind's eye, though, and, truth or not, I couldn't stop now. I told them I was hiding behind the column, sneaking around it to keep out of sight of a guard. I remember that this sounded to me like a strange thing to be doing because this was, after all, *my* house. Yet I knew that my goal was to make my way undetected to a set of stairs that led underground to a chamber where the court magicians kept the tools of their trade.

No one was allowed down there, including me. The magicians felt that they were the only ones who knew how to use these tools. I knew differently. I knew that *I* was the only person who had the ability to use them; the magicians were fooling themselves, or trying to fool the rest of us.

I also knew that among the treasures in the subterranean chamber were golden scepters of various lengths, some as long as six feet. They were crowned with enormous gems, one in particular in a setting of golden prongs. This one had an immense dark-green stone, either an emerald or polished moldavite, something I'd learn more about later.

The next thing I remember, Dr. Weiss was saying, "Okay, let's move to the end of this lifetime."

I went a little further than that. Suddenly I knew that I'd died and left that lifetime. The consciousness I had at that time told me that the power wasn't in the rods at all—it was in *me*, and I took it with me from lifetime to lifetime.

That was the end of my session. From that day until this one, I can't be sure I didn't make up the whole story. While I was on stage, I certainly felt the need to come up with something to say.

After the session was over, many people from the audience told me, "If you'd been out here watching, you'd *know* that you weren't making it up."

Dr. Weiss later told me that while regressed, I'd brought information through that he'd already ascertained for his next book. It was very unlikely that I'd known those things before stepping onto that stage, he said.

I had to agree. And although there was nothing in the "feel" of that experience to tell me that it was real, none of what I'd told him had been in the paper on "Egyptology" I'd written back in the third grade.

✐ ✐ ✐

CHAPTER SIX

The Quest for Explanations

"Recognize what is in your sight,
and that which is hidden from you will become plain to you."
— The Nag Hammadi Library

I figured that someone *had* to know what all these strange occurrences meant. Certainly *my* experiences weren't unique. Someone, somewhere, had to have the answers.

I started, of course, back with the woman on Venice Beach. When she heard about the blisters and bleeding, she admitted that she had no idea what was going on or why. She'd run out of suppositions and New Age platitudes and said it was time I contacted *another* woman, the person who had "taught her and everyone else" how to do this work. She gave me a name and a phone number.

It was too late to call that evening, so I phoned the next day and told this new "teacher" the entire story: the lights coming on, the doors opening, the "people" I sensed in my home and the ones my patients sensed in the office, and my palms blistering and bleeding. I was optimistic about learning something helpful from her. After I finished my story, there was a long silence on the other end of the phone. Then this teacher said, "I don't know of anyone who's ever responded like this. It's *fascinating*." That's all she had to offer.

Apparently, "fascinating" was New Age for "You're on your own, Kiddo." But I wasn't ready to give up. The next month, on the recommendation of a friend, I contacted a world-renowned L.A. psychic. When I set up an appointment to see him, I didn't mention what had been happening to me; I didn't even tell him my last name. I wanted to see if he'd pick up anything on his own and maybe have some idea what was going on with me.

On the day of my appointment, out of breath, lost, and 30 minutes late, I rushed into his condo, plopped down on a chair, and pretended not to notice "the glare." You know, that look mastered by the anally retentive, terminally prompt; the one that causes you to flash back to every lecture you've ever received about being on time, while simultaneously making you question your value as a human being. I was certain that on his days off, he was petitioning Congress to bring back the use of the word *tardy* in our public school system. This reading was shot, I was sure.

The psychic spread his cards in a very businesslike fashion, carefully not displaying a hint of warmth or compassion. He looked at the cards, then looked me straight in the eyes with what was either a slightly quizzical expression or a scowl. "What is it that you do?" he practically demanded.

Now, I don't know about you, but at $100 an hour, I was thinking, *You're the psychic. You tell me.* I refrained from verbalizing my thoughts. "I'm a chiropractor," I replied in a matter-of-fact voice, being careful not to reveal anything that might color my reading.

"Oh, no," he said, "it's much more than that. Something comes out through your hands, and people receive healings. You'll be on television," he continued, "and people will come from all over the country to see you."

This was the *last* thing I expected to hear from this man—especially after the way the session had started out. Well, almost the last thing I expected to hear, because the next thing he told me was that I'd be writing books. "Let me tell you something," I replied with a knowing smile. "If there's one thing I'm sure of, it's that I *won't* be writing any books."

And I meant it. Books and I had never gotten along. By that point in my life, I had read maybe two books, one of which I was still coloring. My favorite pastime had long been watching television. I was, to be blunt, a TV addict.

Oddly enough, after my visit with the psychic, I found myself reading. And reading. My addiction to television had come to an abrupt halt, replaced by, dare I say it, books. I couldn't get enough—Eastern philosophy, life after death, channeled information, even UFO experiences. I read everything, everyone, everywhere.

Bit by bit, my life was being taken over by this strange new energy. At night when I laid down to go to sleep, my legs would vibrate. My hands felt as if they were constantly "on." The bones of my skull would also vibrate, and my ears would buzz. Later I began to hear tones, and on rare occasions, what sounded like voices in choir.

"That's it. I've lost my sanity." I was certain now. Everyone knows that when you go crazy, you hear voices. Mine were singing. In choir yet. I couldn't have a little light humming, a faint vocalist, or even a small chorale group. No, I get The Mormon Tabernacle Choir.

And what about my patients? They were seeing colors: exquisite blues, greens, purples, golds, and whites. Hues of a beauty beyond anything we're familiar with. Although they were able to recognize these colors, they told me that they had never before seen these particular manifestations. I was told by some patients who worked in the film industry that not only do these colors not exist as we know color here on Earth, but even using all their resources and technology, it would be impossible to reproduce them. Hearing this, I flashed back to my mother's life-after-death experience when she spoke of the "indescribable hues and forms" that didn't exist in the world she left behind, and how the sight of them had filled her with wonder.

Manifesting Symptoms

Whether I understood the ultimate source of the energy I was using or not, the healings continued. Even though I wondered about the origins, I rarely questioned the results. If I had, there were probably people I would never have even tried to connect with a healing.

I had made plans to fly across the country at the end of the year (1993) and spend the holidays with Zeida. The night before I left, I was invited to a dinner party. I didn't really want to go, especially since I get pretty neurotic just before a trip—what do I pack, what do I leave, what am I going to forget? Still, I managed to make it to the party.

When I arrived, the host mentioned that one of the guests was in an advanced stage of AIDS. It was clear the moment I saw him: His skin had the grayish pallor that often shows up in the latter stages of the disease, and he was wheeling around an IV morphine drip for the pain and using the stand for balance. He also suffered from a complication called cytomegalovirus, or CMV, which had affected his right eye, completely blurring his vision on that side.

This man was past the point of thinking that his pain would ever be gone, but he really hoped he could at least regain his vision. The host asked if I'd work on him, and I said, "Sure, I'd be happy to." I took him into another room and worked on him for about five minutes, after which he said his pain had almost disappeared.

We both thought that was pretty good progress, and I walked out of the room. A minute or so later, he came out and announced that he could see clearly through both eyes. That was a very exciting moment.

Equally exciting, but in a different way, was when I woke up the next morning and discovered that *my* eye—the left one—had swollen to three times its normal size! For some reason, whenever I temporarily "acquired" someone else's symptoms, it always targeted the opposite side of my body— I don't know why. My eye stayed swollen for about 36 hours.

The blisters and bleeding had been okay with me, but this was something else. I began to wonder, *Am I taking on someone else's illness when I do this energy work? Am I holding on to that illness? Will it set up some kind of a chain response in me afterward?* These thoughts were making me feel a bit uncomfortable.

Then the realization hit me: I didn't *need* to physically manifest other people's problems or symptoms in order for healings to occur—nor did I need these signs to serve as evidence that something real and powerful was going on.

After that revelation, I never had another physical manifestation.

But someone else did.

❧ ❧ ❧

Chapter Seven

The Gift of the Stone

"Any sufficiently advanced technology is indistinguishable from magic."
— from *The Lost Worlds of 2001*, by Arthur C. Clarke

In our culture, January is the start of the year, a time for reflections on the past and resolutions for the future. Looking back on the year 1993, I saw a string of healings that filled me with awe and wonder. Looking forward, I saw . . . *what?* How far would this go? Where was it leading me? I didn't have a clue—at that time, I still hadn't met Gary (from Chapter 1), or experienced the leap of potential his healing was to represent.

Of course, I was playing this entire healing thing by ear—no instruction book, no step-by-step drawings, and not much in the way of advice from acknowledged masters in things "metaphysical." All I could do was continue what I was doing and hope that whatever was bringing this energy to me would do its part as well.

As is often the case, I didn't recognize the next step in the process for what it was when it first occurred. Shortly after I returned to my office following the holidays, one of my patients gave me a little white gift box. I remember feeling that there was something odd about being given a holiday gift *after* the holidays. Although it was the kind of box that might contain a small piece of jewelry, I knew what was going to be inside. Ever since the healings had begun, patients had been bringing me gifts. Everyone thought that I needed something.

"Something" usually fell into one of three categories: (1) books or tapes—I received a lot of those; (2) statues—I've been given every version of Buddha, Moses, Jesus, the Virgin Mary, Krishna, and the archangels you can imagine; and (3) crystals. Crystals come in two sizes: Volkswagen-sized—the sort of thing you have to stand in the corner of a room, assuming the room is large enough—and pocket-sized. People who give pocket-sized crystals take the term *pocket-sized* very seriously. They expect to see that crystal *in your pocket!* There is only one way you can avoid carrying it there, though, and that's if you can figure out the appropriate chakra to hang it over, and get the right colored thread or yarn to dangle it from.

I wasn't going to go that far, so I just put the crystals in my pocket. Pretty soon they were bulging. Every time I bent over to do an adjustment, at least one crystal would fall onto the floor. When I bent over to pick it up, the rose quartz crystals—the only ones that were polished and rounded—would take it upon themselves to leap from my pocket and roll down the hallway like scattering marbles. I'm sure that as some of my patients observed this, they were certain I'd lost my own. So as I opened the little gift box, I expected to find something blue or pink or shimmery . . . but to my surprise, I discovered a strange and irregularly shaped, dark green stone looking almost out of place situated so finely on a bed of cotton. I remember thinking that this was not a particularly attractive piece. It didn't sparkle or reflect light; it was roughly formed. It didn't shine with any beautiful colors, yet instead, was a seemingly unremarkable dark, burnished, mottled, murky, blackish-greenish little "thing." At best, it was similar in both color and texture to an overly ripe Haas avocado. In other words, it didn't fit my concept of a crystal.

"What is it?" I asked.

"Moldavite," came the response.

Hmmm . . . moldavite. Mold. What a lovely name. I guess certain molds can take on colors similar to this one, I thought. *I'll have to remember this for next year's holiday gift giving. Maybe I can find some stones called fungus, too, so that everyone doesn't get the same gift.*

Aware that specific domains of influence are often attributed to specific crystals, I asked about the significance of moldavite.

"Look at the color!" my patient said, as if it could have escaped either my notice or my silent commentary. Ignoring my question and the less-than-enraptured expression on my face, he enthusiastically snatched the stone from my fingers and held it up to the window to allow the light to show through it. I wasn't prepared for what I was about to see. With sunlight entering from behind, this previously opaque-looking stone turned a sheer, diaphanous emerald, spellbindingly provocative in the glow of its translucence.

Again, I put forth my earlier question: "What's it for?"

"Well," my patient answered, "it's far too complicated to explain. Just put it in your pocket, and the next time you're at the Bodhi Tree, you can pick up some material on it."

I pushed the green stone into my pocket without giving it another thought and went on with my day.

I had no idea that my world, which was already wobbling a bit on its axis, was about to turn completely upside-down.

✐ ✐ ✐

Later that day, Fred came to my office. Fred was a patient who'd been seeing me for about a year and a half. On this visit, I adjusted him, then told him to close his eyes and not open them until I said so. I brought my hands up and passed them over his body, as usual—but when I got to his head, it jerked back. His eyes rolled out of sight, his mouth opened, and his tongue began moving in a fashion that was clearly forming vowels. Air was audibly escaping through his mouth.

This was, to say the least, disconcerting. Still, the energy was flowing through my hands, and I thought, *Well, I know he's trying to talk.*

I moved my hands slowly in an attempt to locate an area where the sensation became a little stronger. Gently, I moved one way, then another. Searching. But still there were no words out of Fred, just that pantomime of lips and tongue. It was frustrating. I could tell he was trying to speak, and I really wanted to know what he had to say. I brought my ear closer and closer to his mouth, as if that would help. It didn't.

I was in awe of this situation. Meanwhile, I knew the surrounding rooms were filling up with patients who weren't used to waiting. I was certain everyone was wondering, *What's the doctor doing*? I had to stop working with Fred.

I pulled my hands away—but I didn't know what to do with Fred himself, because his tongue was still moving, and he was continuing to emit sounds bearing the promise of speech. I gently touched him on the chest and said, "Fred, I think we're done." His eyes opened. He looked at me, and I looked at him. He didn't say anything, so *I* didn't say anything. Finally he got up, as if it had been a normal visit, and left.

I decided to just forget about the whole thing and let it go. Like I said, Fred had been a patient of mine for about a year and a half, and up until that day, things had been relatively normal.

But less than a week later, Fred came in for another visit. After the adjustment, I brought my hands up to his head—and boom, it rolled back, his lips parted, his tongue started to move, and, once again, air started audibly escaping.

Although I must admit that I expected something to happen, the intensity caused me to step back. I was speechless.

I'd sort of co-created this day's encounter, because earlier, when I had seen Fred out in the reception room, I'd made a point of moving the other patients through the office ahead of him so that we'd have some uninterrupted time. As soon as the movements I'd seen last time began to appear in Fred on this particular day, I let my hands start feeling for a good, strong connection within his energy—a place where I could do whatever might amplify this behavior.

Finally, Fred started to speak.

Now, when most of us talk, we simply open our mouths and a voice comes out—no big surprise. But to hear a voice form itself out of the ethers is a little . . . unsettling. The broken hiss of air I'd heard last time began to evolve into words. The voice that carried them started out as a ragged, high-pitched squeal: *"We are here to tell you . . ."* the voice deepened *". . . to continue doing what you are doing . . ."* the voice went on in a jerky, choppy way. *"What you are doing . . . is bringing light and information onto the planet."*

As Fred spoke, his voice changed, gradually dropping down the scale from a squeal to a deep, resonant boom, yet the phrasing remained oddly mechanical, almost as if the source of this communication had to learn to utilize Fred's voice box. Still, everything he said was clear and compelling.

By this time, all the adjustment rooms had filled up again with patients. That made for a significant number of people. And my adjustment rooms had no doors—there was nothing to keep this strange voice from traveling throughout the office.

Still, I didn't want to let Fred go yet. I wondered if I had the type of personality that could say, "Pardon me, Mr. Voice from the Universe, who traveled so far to communicate with me, but right now isn't convenient. Might you come back at a better time? Seven-thirty would be nice."

It turned out that I couldn't go quite that far, but I did start pushing a bit. "How can I speak with you again?" I asked Fred's voice.

"You may find me in your heart," it said.

That's not an answer; that's a Hallmark card! I wanted this voice again. "Well," I said, "might I be able to reach you through another person?"

The response was vague.

"Might I be able to reach you through this person again?" I asked.

Another noncommittal response. I wasn't about to let it off this easily. So I pushed and pushed and pushed. Finally, the voice said, *"All right. You may speak to me through this person again."*

I touched Fred lightly on his chest, where I had before, and said, "Fred, I think we're done now." He opened his eyes—and shot up off the table and over against the wall, where he stood blocking the telephone. He later told me that he was sure I was going to call a mental hospital and have him taken away. Although he couldn't remember most of what had come out of his mouth, he'd been aware of what had occurred—in principle, at least. He confessed that he'd done this before. He'd only told two people about it and didn't want anyone else to know.

He had noticed the voice starting to speak through him during our previous session, but he thought he'd controlled it and that I hadn't been aware of anything. This time he'd lost control almost immediately, and the voice came through. Fred didn't care for this lack of control at all. He felt that he wasn't in charge of what came out of his own mouth, explaining that it bothered him because he couldn't coherently understand what he was saying either. He described the process like this: He heard one word, and then a second word, and then a third word, but by the time he got to the fourth word, he'd forgotten the first one. It also bothered him that he couldn't put the thoughts together in his own mind.

I assured him that I'd heard of things such as channeling and/or speaking in tongues before, and I figured, well, it's interesting to know someone who does this. I chalked it up as a "Fred" thing.

But a day or two later, it happened again—*with three different patients!* One after another, their heads jerked back, their eyes rolled upward, their lips parted, their tongues moved, and air audibly escaped from their mouths. I was not going to sit around and wait for a double-blind, randomized study. *I knew that on their next visit, they were going to speak.* I wanted answers, and I wanted them now.

The Golden Eye

At this point, I returned to the psychic who had told me about my hands. After all, he *was* reputable. He did readings for royalty in the Middle East, the Reagan White House, and more than a handful of celebrities sought his counsel. I phoned him and explained everything that was happening.

He listened carefully, then said, "Well, I don't know what it is."

This was not confidence-instilling.

"Go to this French woman in Beverly Hills," he told me. "She's studied these things. She can probably help you, if anyone can. Her name is Claude." (Don't ask me why it wasn't Claudine or Claudette; I don't know.)

So I went to see Claude. I figured I'd go in, hold my hands near her, and let her feel what was coming through. Then, in my imagined scenario, she'd explain what it was, I'd gain some clarity, and I could continue with my life.

It seemed that I was the only one who had this expectation. Claude brought me in, sat me down on her sofa, and placed a crystal in each of my hands. Then she displayed a giant piece of poster board with a star drawn on it. Every section of the star was a different color. As if that weren't enough, she'd glued weird little eyes all over the thing, evidently for effect.

She told me to look at the star and the colors, then close my eyes. She started to take me through basic color visualization. This was something I was definitely not in the mood for. I had something *real* going on in my life; if I'd wanted to imagine my own explanations for it, I could have stayed at home and done so. But there I was.

Holding the crystals, I closed my eyes. Claude said, "Now, picture blue. Everything is blue."

I don't know about you, but when I close my eyes, the only color I see is charcoal. But I tried.

"Blue," she said. "Everything is blue."

I'm trying.

"Now visualize red."

Red, I thought.

"Green."

Green.

"Yellow."

Yellow.

"Orange."

Orange.

"Now, picture gold. Everything is gold," Claude said. "Golden sky. Golden ground. Golden mountain. Golden waterfall."

Okay, the whole world's gold.

"Stand under the golden waterfall," she continued. "Feel the golden water falling on you."

This woman's really pushing the envelope, I thought to myself.

"Now picture this golden eye, a giant golden eye up in the sky. You're going to ask this eye questions."

That was all I needed to hear. I opened my eyes and looked at her. "And *how* is it going to answer me? It's an *eye*."

"Just close your eyes, and I'll tell you what questions to ask."

"Fine," I said, and closed my eyes.

"Ask the eye how many strands of DNA you have."

Nervous and frustrated, I opened my eyes once more and looked at her. "I *know* how many strands of DNA I have; I'm a *doctor*." I proceeded to explain RNA and DNA to her, describing single strands, double strands, and the double helix formation.

She listened patiently. Then, as if nothing I had said contained even a hint of relevance, she resumed. "Ask the eye."

So I sat there and closed my eyes for the third time, trying to figure out how I was going to get out of this nonsense. How was I going to ask this eye (which I couldn't see) a question that it couldn't answer anyway because it *was* an eye, not a mouth—the answer to which, I already knew, was "two"— and get out of this woman's apartment without appearing really rude? Suddenly, I opened my eyes and looked at her, plain as day, as I heard myself say: "I have three. There are twelve strands of DNA. Twelve."

Now, no one had told me this was a two-part question, so I had no idea why I answered that way. Especially since what I said went against everything I had consciously known up to that point.

"Oh," Claude said. "You're a Pleiadian."

"Oh?" I asked. "What's a Pleiadian?"

She explained that the Pleiades is a system of seven stars, clearly visible from Earth. (As soon as I got home, I looked it up, and she was right.)

Claude went on to explain that at one point, Earth was considered a way-station of light and information for travelers throughout the universe. They would stop here to relax, rejuvenate, and access information, as Earth was considered to be a living library. The people running the planet at the time were Pleaidians. At some point, there arose a struggle, and an ideological and political schism formed between two Pleiadian factions. Each group wanted to take control—not just over the other group, but over the planet as a whole. But since the members of each faction were of equal strength and intelligence, all they could foresee was a future of continual battle to attain a position of superiority. This was not acceptable to either, so they maintained a sort of truce until the scientists of one group found a way to disconnect 10 of the original 12 strands of DNA from the members of the other group. We are said to be the descendants of those modified Pleaidians. *Who knew?*

Yet, those of us who supposedly have our third strand—who are closer, in theory, to our progenitors—have come back to bring light and information onto this planet—which is exactly what Fred had told me—or rather, channeled to me.

Now, I'm not telling you that I'm a Pleaidian, nor am I saying that Pleaidians actually exist. All I'm suggesting at this point is that you continue to follow this story.

Giving Myself Over

I went over to the Bodhi Tree, and while I was there, I decided to do some research on that little green stone in my pocket. From what I discovered, moldavite is not an Earth crystal; it's a meteorite that fell to Earth over Eastern Europe approximately 15 million years ago. It's supposed to have the ability to open up communication with (depending on your source of information) angels, entities, and beings from other dimensions. Is this true? Does this stone really hold the capacity for interdimensional communication? *I don't know.* What I *do* know is that I put the stone in my pocket, and the channeling started.

I was faced with a choice. Things had been getting stranger in my life by the minute, even before Fred brought the first voice through. Where would this lead me? Ultimately, I had to make a decision about whether or not to continue along this new and unfamiliar path. What was I doing? Was this good? Was this bad? Was I listening to the "right" voices? How could I be sure about the intentions of whatever source lay behind all this?

My initial response was to ask everyone who I thought should know, such as healers, mediums, psychics, et cetera. They were fairly unanimous. These people felt that, unless and until I was able to determine the source of these voices, I should stay away from them.

I was left, then, in a real quandary. How was this done? Do you ask the voice? Doesn't that leave you with the age-old dilemma of "If it's an honest voice, it will tell you the truth, and if it's a dishonest voice, it won't." Either way, you get the same answer. Do I shoot it with a silver bullet? Wear a necklace made of garlic? Buy a large cross? I found it very difficult to believe that this voice (or *these* voices) would take the time and trouble to make their way through the universe simply to orchestrate some grand and cosmic joke.

I realized that my emotions surrounding this process were now running a more narrow gamut: apprehension to alarm to panic. It became clear that all of the well-intended advice I had been receiving had one unifying thread: fear. And I realized that there was an even bigger choice I had to make: whether I was willing to base the (potentially) largest decision of my life on fear. I was *not*. The answer was both suddenly apparent and incontrovertible. I had decided that I was going to give myself over to whatever it was that was coming through me.

🕸 🕸 🕸

❧ Chapter Eight ❧

Insights: Present and Future

"And away we go!"
— Jackie Gleason

Back in the office, the three patients who had "spoken" in voices, as Fred had done, returned for their next appointments. Just as I'd predicted, *boom*—one after the other, their heads flew back, their eyes rolled upward, their tongues began to move, air audibly began to escape from their mouths . . . and what did they say?

"We are here to tell you to continue doing what you are doing. What you are doing is bringing light and information onto the planet." The exact same phrases Fred had spoken. But these patients didn't know Fred. For that matter, they didn't know one another.

Two of the patients added another phrase: *"What you are doing is reconnecting strands."*

The third patient said something slightly different: *"What you are doing is reconnecting strings."*

The next time Fred came in, he told me he'd been doing some automatic writing—and there, in his own handwriting, the last line (in reference to me) read: *"What he is doing is reconnecting strings."*

Two days later, more patients began to utter these phrases. I carefully interviewed them afterward, and discovered that, except for Fred, none of them had ever done anything of this sort before.

But for whatever reason, they had been chosen as vehicles for these voices, and no matter what other words came out of their mouths, they all repeated these same six phrases:

1. *We are here to tell you to continue doing what you are doing.*
2. *What you are doing is bringing light and information onto the planet.*
3. *What you are doing is reconnecting strands.*
4. *What you are doing is reconnecting strings.*
5. *You must know that you are a master.*
6. *We've come because of your reputation.*

I thought, *Okay, What you're doing is bringing light and information onto the planet . . .* so I kept waiting to receive this information. . . .

Yet it didn't seem to be forthcoming.

All right, then, I thought—*information such as what? How to grow giant fruit? How to put up an interplanetary defense system? How to build flying saucers?* I still had no idea what was going on.

Fade Out

I kept waiting for the promises of the phrases to be fulfilled, but in April of 1994, something began to change. First, the voices appeared to be struggling to get through. The ease with which people had involuntarily broken into channel was diminishing, and the channelings themselves became less frequent. In fact, they took a sudden, drastic drop.

And then it was over. Except for Fred, there were no more channelings, no more voices.

Prior to this, I had on occasion wondered if the whole thing had been a joke. Had my receptionist been selecting patients at random and saying to them, "Look, here are your lines. Don't let the doctor see the script."

Now the voices were gone, and I knew that it had *not* been a joke. Nothing about it could have been more real. I felt a sense of emptiness. These strange occurrences had, after all, become the center of my life. How could they be over?

By the time the channelings had ceased, the six phrases had been given to me independently by more than 50 people. Remember that, aside from Fred, none of those people had ever channeled before—and some of them were so unnerved by the experience that they never returned to my office. Given this evidence, as well as the remarkably consistent descriptions of various entities, it became clear to me that during a healing session, *there was someone other than myself and the patient in the room.* And that other person, or "being," was speaking through the body of the person on the table. I don't know if the "channelers" were like radios picking up signals beaming in from all over the universe, or if they were all getting the same signal from one central source, but I suppose it doesn't matter. The message had come through loud and clear.

This could explain why the channelings finally came to a halt: *I'd gotten the point.* There was no way that anyone, even I, could deny that something real and profound was going on here. Although I still craved the reinforcement of the channeled entities, the source had decided I'd had all I needed. It was time to stop looking for more and to allow myself to see what I'd already been given.

When you go through an experience such as this, you *know* you're connecting with something from somewhere else. I quickly let go of the practical joke theory and waited. But when this mysterious "information" I was supposed to get still didn't arrive, the emptiness deepened. What had I done to cause the voices to abandon me?

However, I still felt the sensations in my hands, and I continued to work with patients just as I had been doing. The healings went on. In fact, it was during this time that Gary came to see me and we had what I would consider the first "major" healing. So despite my despair over not receiving what I thought was the promised information, I continued to work with patients and move my hands over them just as I had been doing. Now and then, their facial muscles—especially those around their mouths—would start to move, but they never really spoke.

Still, when they came out of their sessions, these patients would tell me they'd "seen" things. Often, the reports were similar: certain shapes, certain colors . . . and certain people. Call them angels, guides, entities, spirits, whatever works for you. But whatever they were, based on the descriptions I got, they usually looked just like real people.

Insights and Validations

At roughly the same time I "got" the insight that I had been given a profound gift, and decided to accept it, I received a call from the producers of a TV show called *The Other Side,* which featured stories about all kinds of paranormal occurrences. They'd heard about me and wanted me to appear on the program. I agreed, and took Gary along to tell his story.

After the show aired in the middle of 1995, people from all over the country started to visit my office. A woman named Michele came down from Seaside, Oregon. When she was lying on the table, I moved my hands over her and watched her involuntary muscular responses as the energy flowed. That's all I saw. But when I was finished, she opened her eyes and said, "I saw a woman. I think she's a guardian angel. And she told me that I would be better, that I would be healed."

Michele's Story

Michele was diagnosed with chronic fatigue syndrome and fibromyalgia. Her symptoms were so severe that many of the doctors who had examined her thought that she had other complications as well. This led to an array of painkillers and other medications. Her life was a constant cycle of pain and exhaustion. Little things such as washing the dishes, cooking dinner, or even just getting out of bed each morning became major undertakings and were sometimes impossible to complete. Her husband had to carry her into a hot shower up to four times a night just to ease her pain. She couldn't eat, and her weight dropped to 87 pounds.

One evening when everyone in her house was sleeping, she swallowed several handfuls of pain pills, haphazardly mixing them all together. As the drugs took effect, she found herself praying: "Please, God, help me. I can't live like this, but I don't want to leave my boys." She felt that she simply couldn't be sick any longer, but didn't know where to turn for help.

She must have fallen asleep on the floor, because the next thing she recalls, she was awakened by the morning sun coming in through the bathroom window. Feeling sick and exhausted, she dragged herself to the sofa. Lying there, she turned on the TV—a talk show was on. I was being interviewed along with a panel of medical doctors. The discussion was about my patients and how so many of them had been healed of unusual afflictions. She watched as I explained that the healings seemed to be brought about by a "Higher Power," which somehow came through me. Michele called the television station for my number.

Her first session began in a quiet room with dim lights and a soothing atmosphere. I lightly placed one finger above her heart, and she immediately fell into a light sleep. I then held my hands over and above her head. A warmth entered and surrounded her body. The energy level in the room became very intense as her eyes began to roll side-to-side, and her fingers adopted an almost marionette-like motion. She simultaneously experienced a continuous, involuntary movement of her right knee.

At one point, I left her alone for a moment. When I returned, Michele said she had the strongest feeling that someone else had come into the room. She had heard the soft voice of a woman, and the woman tried to tell Michele her name. It was difficult for her to make it out clearly, as the communication came in what could only be described as "almost" a voice. At first, Michele thought that the woman had a bit of an attitude, but then it became clear that this woman was just frustrated that Michele couldn't quite understand her.

The woman told Michele that she was her guardian angel, and that her name was something like Parsley, or Parcel. She eventually heard the name: Parsillia. Then the angel said the strangest thing. She said to Michele: *You will be healed. And you are to go on television and talk about it.* This was, to my way of thinking at the time, not something an angel would say. Just the same, it wasn't my place to make editorial comments. The physicians had done all that they could for Michele, but Parsillia's presence had told her that her life was now beginning again.

After that session, Michele's appetite returned.

Her second session, the next day, was just as dramatic. The guardian angel came back. Again, several areas of Michele's body became hot, then relaxed and got warm. She became so warm that even her legs turned a bright pink. Once again, Parsillia told Michele several times that she was being healed. In fact, Michele had so much energy after her second session that she decided to go shopping with her mom. While they were out together, her mother actually had to tell Michele to slow down. This was a pleasant shock for both of them.

During Michele's third and fourth sessions, the angel told her that she was healed and would gradually notice other changes. Michele saw flowers with colors she had never seen before, and she felt happiness all around her. She instantly understood that everyone had a purpose. She was also told to spend more time with her sons.

For Michele, life returned to normal. Her weight went back up, she started exercising daily, and she started to work full-time in her own business.

A Little Knowledge

Before Michele came to my office, a number of patients had described seeing human-appearing angels or beings. Yet, never had I heard a story as detailed and elaborate as hers. *Well,* I thought, *what do you expect? Look what you're doing—you're* bound *to attract the kind of people who think they see angels.*

A month or two after Michele's healing, a man from Beverly Hills visited my office. He wasn't ill; it was just that he'd heard about what was going on in my office and wanted to experience it.

After his session, he opened his eyes and said, "I saw this woman, and she said to tell you she was here, that you'd know who she was. She seemed to have a bit of an attitude, but I could tell she was just frustrated that she couldn't clearly communicate her name. It was something like Parsley. Then she said to me, 'If you have a healing, will you go on television and talk about it?'"

I was stunned. Who was this Parsley character, the Angel of Public Relations? No—she was *confirmation.*

I never saw the man again. He didn't know any of my other patients— and yet he knew about the angel with the funny name.

Things were just warming up.

A woman flew in from New Jersey with her daughter, an 11-year-old with scoliosis, a curvature of the spine. After the daughter's session, she opened her eyes and looked quite surprised. As had become the norm, I asked, "What went on? What did you notice?"

"Well," she said, "I saw this tiny little multicolored parrot, and he told me his name was George. Then he wasn't a parrot at all; he wasn't even a life form."

Life form, she said. Her words. An 11-year-old girl.

"Then," the little girl added, "he just became my friend."

Not long after that, a man—a full-grown adult—came in for a session. When it was over, he said, "I found myself at this statue, this marble outdoor statue, standing around an old Roman or Greek pond centuries ago. And as I looked down toward my right hand, I saw this tiny little multicolored parrot. He told me his name was George. And then he wasn't a parrot at all; then he just became my friend."

Except for the omission of "life form," it was the same story as the girl's—verbatim.

I felt even more vulnerable than usual when I decided to explain what was going on in my life to my cousin, whose opinion I valued. I drew in a deep breath and braced myself as I heard phrases such as "my palm blistered," "another time it bled," and "my patients are losing consciousness and speaking in voices other than their own" sputter from my mouth in an awkwardly self-conscious cadence.

"If it were anyone other than you," she said after I finished, "I wouldn't have believed them. But I know that you wouldn't make this up. I've known you all your life. You're too grounded." Hearing this from my cousin who used to baby-sit me when I was a kid, I suddenly realized that I had no idea how I came across to people—or that others' perceptions of me were so different from my own. I had no idea that so many people would tell me that they believed me when I told them what was happening *"because* it was you," *"because* you're so grounded," *"because* you're so real," *"because* you're so skeptical."

Grounded. Real. Skeptical. I knew I was a little skeptical—if only because I didn't really believe them when they told me they thought I was grounded. I mean, I thought of myself as grounded (at times, anyway), but I certainly didn't realize I was perceived that way.

Despite this reinforcement, it took me a while to tell my parents what was going on in my life. I'll never forget my father's response: "Don't ever leave that office!" As if the angels, like the ghost who used to haunt the Melrose Place building, were somehow locked into that particular address.

Luckily, these healings, including the experiential aspect of them such as the angels and the colors, occurred just as successfully when I traveled, so I knew that if these entities really were assigned to Melrose Place, at least they were capable of checking my schedule and arranging their own transportation to my destination.

Not that I needed to travel that much. Not with the way people were coming to see me.

The Courage to Step Forth

The healings were getting more amazing all the time. And yet, while the results were rewarding, the results in and of themselves didn't seem to be enough for me. I still wanted to know *why* the healings were happening. What did this phenomenon mean? Where was it coming from? My quest for understanding was never-ending.

I decided to attend a three-day seminar given by Deepak Chopra, M.D. (Dr. Chopra is, of course, one of the major figures in the current synthesis of medicine and spirituality, including the melding of quantum physics and ancient wisdom.) Most of the audience members at the seminar consisted of doctors and other professionals. Perhaps because of my peculiar success with Brian Weiss, I thought I would be able to find a moment to ask Dr. Chopra a quiet little question that might render some insight into what was going on with me and these healings. I noticed that there were microphones on stands here and there in the room, which appeared to be intended for audience participation.

As the seminar progressed, no one on the staff made reference to either the microphones or the possibility of audience interaction. Time went by. Finally, just before the lunch break on the second day, I couldn't contain myself any longer. I raised my hand and asked Dr. Chopra if he would, at any point, be entertaining questions.

Dr. Chopra surprised me by asking a question of his own: "Do you *have* a question?"

"Yes, I do," I said.

"Go up to the microphone, then, and ask it."

As I took the seemingly endless walk toward the nearest microphone, I became aware of the ever-increasing volume of my footsteps in contrast with the sudden silence in the room, woven from very loud intertwining thoughts:

Who is *this person?*
Why does he *get to ask a question?*
I *wanted to ask a question.*
I could be eating lunch right now.
And the proverbial . . .
This had better be good.

As I approached the microphone, Dr. Chopra prompted me, "So what is your question?"

I didn't know. I hadn't formulated it yet. To make matters worse, I suddenly realized that, without Dr. Chopra knowing some of the background of what had been going on in my life since August of 1993, it wouldn't be possible for me to ask my question even after I'd figured out what it was. So, as succinctly as possible, I tried to quickly explain what had happened— including the voices, the bleeding, and the blistering. I hoped that by the end of this introduction, the perfect question would make itself apparent to me.

At the end of my synopsis, what I found myself saying was, "Please don't think I don't know what this sounds like, because I do. But I wonder if you have any insights or advice?"

It wasn't even a question exactly. I watched as Dr. Chopra leaned forward from where he stood on the stage.

Then he asked, "What's your last name?"

I took a startled half-step back. "Pearl!" I blurted.

He nodded. "I've heard of you." He looked out over the room. "And I want everyone here to know that everything this man has just said is true." In front of everyone in the room, he invited me to come down to The Chopra Center for Well Being in La Jolla (near San Diego) to do some research.

Then came his advice: "Remain childlike." Two words that meant so much.

I'll never forget it.

The Beginnings of Research

As I'd been told to expect, more and more television producers started asking me to appear on their shows. Fox TV wanted to interview me during a major convention up in the San Francisco area, along with others such as Dr. Andrew Weil, the white-bearded doctor and bestselling author of *Eating Well for Optimum Health,* who wages a highly visible war in favor of consolidating "traditional" and "alternative" medicine.

Before I left Los Angeles for the seminar, and completely out of the blue, I got an e-mail from my parents. They told me something rather surprising: My father and Dr. Weil's father had both run on the same local political ticket and had served on various boards together in my hometown some years back. My parents and his had, in fact, been friends. Somehow, this little piece of information had never come up before now.

Then my mother told me something very touching about Dr. Weil's father, Dan. The story was this: Back in the early 1980s, my father had quadruple-bypass surgery. While he was recovering, Dan Weil, a warm and compassionate man, sent a letter—not to him, but to my mother. The letter pointed out that during such trying times, most people send cards to the person in the hospital, and we forget that it's often the person left at home who needs the most support. His letter was filled with kindness and encouragement, and was something my parents never forgot. Dan Weil had since passed on, and my parents thought that his son might appreciate hearing how his father had touched their lives. They wrote Dr. Weil a letter and asked me to pass it on to him.

Andrew Weil happened to be in the hotel lobby at the same time I was checking into the seminar. I introduced myself and gave him the letter. He asked if he might have the letter his father wrote to show to his mother. We exchanged a polite word or two, and that was the last I thought I'd see of the doctor.

That night, I received a call from the woman who had not only arranged the Fox interviews, but who was also conducting them. She'd been in a car accident the previous week and had broken some ribs, so she had to walk with a cane, and her broken ribs allowed her only the shallowest of breaths. She could hardly speak—not the most ideal circumstances for interviewing people. She asked if I'd give her a session that evening. I told her it would be my pleasure. It turned out to be more than that, however. It turned out to be one more piece of the synchronicity puzzle.

The next morning, I showed up for my interview and discovered that Dr. Weil was scheduled for the time slot next to mine. It so happened that he, the interviewer, and I all crossed paths. As Dr. Weil came in, the interviewer was thanking me for her session and explaining how she no longer needed her cane, explaining that she was now able to breathe deeply and fully enough to conduct the interviews.

Dr. Weil asked what I'd done. After I explained what little I could, he invited me to come to the University of Arizona and address the Fellows attending his Program of Integrated Medicine (PIM). The invitation was an honor that I happily accepted. This led me to Gary E. R. Schwartz, Ph.D., who runs the Human Energy Systems Department at the University of Arizona. He, along with his wife, Linda G.S. Russek, Ph.D., is also the author of *The Living Energy Universe*, which presents the idea that everything, at every level of existence, is alive, remembers, and evolves. This book endeavors to explain not only some of the greatest enigmas of conventional science, but also mysteries such as homeopathy, survival after death, and psychic abilities.

Dr. Schwartz invited me to return to the university to do research on the healings. I accepted.

Crossroads

Things were moving faster and faster. It was tempting to just continue being swept along, but could I really do that? There were other considerations. I'd spent a significant part of my life creating a successful practice, and all this involvement with "healing energy" and "channeled spirits" hadn't done it a bit of good. For one thing, as I mentioned earlier, some of the patients who channeled had been so shaken up by the experience that they simply never came back. But that wasn't the worst of it. Imagine visiting your chiropractor and hearing bizarre-sounding voices coming from the adjacent rooms. It could make you wonder . . .

On many occasions, I've said to myself, "You must be nuts. You've got mortgage payments, car payments—and a large practice that you need to maintain in order to make ends meet. Just stick to chiropractic."

But that wasn't what the entities meant when they said, *We are here to tell you to continue doing what you are doing,* and I knew it. So I continued to do this new "thing." Even when there were gaps or declines in the healings, I continued to work with the energy anyway. I kept doing what I was doing.

🦢 🦢 🦢

Why me? I couldn't help but wonder. I'm told that this is a question of ego, yet when your life turns upside down and the basic tenets of reality you've accepted since birth no longer apply, it becomes a difficult question not to ask.

I found myself contemplating the phrases again. *What you are doing is bringing light and information onto the planet.* Clearly, this meant there was something more going on than *just* "healing" people, at least in the usual sense of the word *heal.* And, *You must know that you are a master* had pretty strong connotations, too. The problem was, I just couldn't think of myself as a particularly good candidate for prophet status. I liked to drink, I liked to eat, I liked to have fun, I liked to stay out all night. Yes, it's true that my fascination—in some cases, obsession—with these pastimes had dwindled a lot since that day on Venice Beach, and even more so since the day I'd stood at the window of my office and watched Gary struggling up the steps. Yet surely other people appeared to be far more "worthy," so *that* didn't make sense.

Part of the reason might be that I have such a big mouth: I'm willing to go out there and speak about these things. Also, it might be because I seem to be able to bridge a gap. I clean up nicely and have the ability to present myself fairly lucidly in hospitals and universities where I am frequently invited to address physicians, educators, and researchers on a topic that is, to say the least, "out there." Also, I find that I have no trouble speaking with those who profess to be metaphysical spiritualists. While these two groups who seem to exist on opposite ends of the spectrum tend to spend most of their time either shouting at or trying to ignore one another, I seem to have the ability to take the hand of each and introduce them as people who might have something interesting to offer in the way of exchange.

Or maybe, in the end, I'd been chosen long before I was capable of thinking about it. Maybe I'd been selected on the night I was born and my mother was reborn, the night the magnificent *Light* told my mother she had a job to do: raising me. Maybe I'd been assigned my future job right then. And quite possibly what's happening now is that I'm *reconnecting* to it.

Healer, Teach Thyself

Gary's healing and the television appearance that followed it were turning points in my life. All of a sudden, I found myself surrounded by two types of people: those who wanted healings, and those who wanted me to teach them how to *do* healings. Eventually, teaching organizations of various kinds began to approach me with the same request.

"You *can't* teach it," I replied. I mean, how could anyone? Nobody had taught it to *me*. It just . . . arrived.

"Sure you can," came the inevitable buck-up-and-put-your-nose-to-the-grindstone response. "Lots of people teach healing. There are books and tapes on the subject in all the stores." Then they'd rattle off a list of authors and titles, many of which you're probably familiar with. But as I read through the books and listened to the tapes, I found that, essentially, the instructions all boiled down to something along these lines: "Place your client on their back (or in a chair). Stand on a specific side of the person [your book will be happy to tell you which side is best], place your right hand here and your left hand there, then move your right hand up to where your left hand is and move your left hand farther up the body to another place. . . ." [Don't worry. Your book will not only specify where to place your hands each step of the way, it will also tell you in which direction to face and in which direction to walk. If that's not enough, it will even tell you what to think while you're doing all this.]

This, I realized, was not healing. It was a tango. And the world did not need another dance class.

There didn't seem to be much help offered up in the myriad seminars on the subject, either—big or small, inexpensive, expensive, or exorbitantly expensive. Let's talk about some of those seminars. To be a healer, you don't need to spend $40,000 on a four-year course studying other healers and hypnotists through the ages. To paraphrase Dr. Reginald Gold, a chiropractor and present-day philosopher, that doesn't make you a *healer*, that makes you an *historian*. In other words, most healing schools don't teach healing at all; they teach the history of certain healers. You'll learn what this healer thought, what that healer thought, and if you're particularly unlucky, you'll learn what *you're* supposed to think, too.

I entered into each new structured educational experience—be it book, tape, or seminar—in a state of expectancy, only to find that I was being served up the same warmed-over bowl of spiritual oatmeal. The one I was given had been room-temperature for so long that it was forming a skin on top. Yet during seminars, half the attendees sat there entranced, as if pearls of newfound knowledge were being laid before them. The other half sat there smiling and nodding in agreement. Not the quiet little nod they might give if they were in a room by themselves reading a book or listening to someone on the radio; these were big, showy, oversized nods designed to demonstrate to others that the instructor was saying something they knew all along, and that somehow their concurrence would validate them to everyone else in the room. (Remember, the quest for spiritual growth does not always preclude the game of one-upmanship.)

Bolstered by the mounting evidence from these experiences, I became even more secure in my earlier statement: *You can't teach healing.* And guess what? I still believe that.

So why am I writing this book? Because while I was focused on my search to discover whether (how?) healing could be taught at all, I failed to notice a phenomenon of increasing frequency that had been occurring right there in my office. You see, a growing number of people who had been in for healings were phoning in, usually after their initial session with me, to say that when they got home, they found that their televisions, stereos, lights, refrigerators—electrical appliances of all kinds—were turning themselves on and off. Repeatedly.

Rarely was there a permanent stoppage, although you might wonder, because the appliances might shut off or fail to work for periods ranging from a few minutes to several days. Usually, the larger the item, the longer the downtime. It was as if the appliances had taken on lives of their own. The experience felt, to most people, like they were being communicated with somehow. I think that's accurate. I'm of the mind that it's someone saying, "Hello. I really *am* here. We really *do* exist."

These same people would then report that they felt something happening in their hands—strange sensations: warm and electrical, or cool and breezy. They'd go on to explain that when they held their hands near someone who was in discomfort or had an ailment, quite often that person's symptoms would diminish or disappear entirely: psoriasis cleared up, asthma went away, chronic wounds healed. Often these results would occur overnight or on the spot. On and on, the stories and phone calls continued to come in. It was out of this that I realized that although healing really can't be "taught," the ability to heal can, somehow, be "communicated" to people. What can be taught, then, is the recognition and the refining of this ability (which I'm attempting to do through the writing of this book).

I finally called one of the organizations who'd been courting me and agreed to teach a class. I told them to gather the people and we'd give it a go.

The evening of the class arrived. Somewhere along the way, driving in the peak of L.A.'s famous rush-hour traffic, I decided not to use any notes. As I entered the room, everyone was already in their seats. Twenty-five people. I hadn't expected that big of a turnout. I walked to the front of the room, pushed the stool and podium out of the way, and, kicking off my shoes, sat cross-legged on the folding table, which for some reason had been placed in front of the room and was gracious enough not to collapse. "I know that you've all come to hear what I've got to say tonight," I said, "and I can't wait to find out what it is myself."

I began with the story of what happened to me in August of 1993, took questions, then "activated" each attendee's hands. I taught them how to play with (or work with, if you prefer) these new energy frequencies—and, after telling them to call me if anything interesting occurred, I released a group of new "healers" onto an unsuspecting planet.

After that, my phone rang off the hook. Again, *who knew?*

Who's the Student Now?

So here I am. The journey has been long and strange and exciting and a bit scary at times, but I think I'm where I'm supposed to be at this point. It's ironic, when you think about it: The terrible student, the one who couldn't hold still, the kid who cut class whenever he could and antagonized the faculty at every opportunity—had become a teacher himself.

The rest of this book is a part of that process. In conducting seminars over the years, I've discovered that, with a fairly minimal amount of instruction, people can connect with this energy and use it in the way it wants to be used.

In a sense, learning to use these energies *is* sort of like mastering the tango. You can manage it by looking at diagrams in a book if you must—but the learning curve is much shorter, and the results better, if you watch a video instead. Yet a video is still not as effective as going to a dance studio and getting hands-on instruction from a qualified teacher.

The same applies here. The remainder of this book will give you a lot of information imparted through words. More of it, however, will be imparted by something *other than* words—whether you want to call it encoding, vibration, or anything else. And yes, you can begin the shift and accommodation of carrying the energy after reading this, because, to varying degrees, the ability to hold and utilize these new frequencies is imparted to those who come in contact with them through the written word, as well as through other forms of media. No, it isn't the same as one-on-one, yet it's a powerful beginning.

✵ ✵ ✵

PART II

Reconnective Healing and What It Means

"The straight lines of time are actually threads of a web extending to infinity."
— from *Living this Moment, Sutras for Instant Enlightenment*

❧ CHAPTER NINE ❧

Tell Me More

"There is a need for a reconciliation of religion and science, just as it is necessary to reconcile intuition and reason, experience and knowledge."
— Dr. Jonas Salk

A s I've described, after my second session with the woman on Venice Beach and the events that followed, I became devoted to learning about what was happening to me. The fact that I willingly started reading books says a lot, but I didn't stop there. Apart from the "experts," "sensitives," and "psychics" I visited—and those who visited me—I asked questions of anyone and everyone whom I thought might be able to offer the slightest hint of insight into what was going on: church leaders, rabbis, Kabbalists, gurus—you name it.

For the most part, what I discerned was that nobody really "knew." At least, nobody in *this* world did. Or, they might know bits and pieces, but not the whole thing. Or, they might have confused my experiences with something they had read about or been taught, but which didn't actually apply here. The most common situation I ran into was that, instead of actually *looking* at this phenomenon, people wanted to explain it from within the comfortable parameters of their specific faith or belief system. They wanted to somehow force it or squeeze it into a box too small, too constrained, too limited to hold.

I had to know more, and I wanted it to come from someone who saw the big picture. I wanted direct conversation with these *angels*, these *beings*. Try as I might, this didn't seem to occur, and I'll tell you, it was more than a bit frustrating. I had observed and listened to my patients enough by now to know that the angels were real. They were *seeing* the angels, *hearing* them, *smelling* their scents—that is, everyone was *but me*. To say I felt left out is a definite understatement. So, as often as I could, I tried to get these beings to communicate, indirectly at least, through Fred.

I want you to know that I don't buy into things simply because they're flattering or sound nice. I don't really care for the term *New Age*. I have serious doubts about many of the people who claim to have "special" and "unique" supernatural gifts, especially when, for all intents and purposes, it appears that many of them are presenting themselves that way merely in an attempt to stand out from the crowd, to get some public acclaim, or to compensate for certain feelings of inferiority. I don't see auras, and I'm not a psychic. So, as far as "channelers" go, let's face it—you don't have to be Linda Blair to moan and shake and speak in a voice that sounds like an old-fashioned record being played at variable speeds.

On the other hand, when more than 50 people who have never met utter the exact same words and, unsolicited, report that they've been witness to the exact same never-before-heard-of entities . . . well, at that point it becomes unreasonable *not* to accept the fact that something authentic is happening.

But what exactly *is* occurring? Where is the healing energy coming from in the first place? Who's sending it? How is it doing what it's doing?

The entities were willing to speak about most things, yet the channelings were only one source of information. Ultimately, I would discover another source of information, one that dwelled deep inside. (Sometimes bravery is going deep inside yourself and trusting what you bring back out . . . but that's another story.)

What I've come to call The Reconnection (a name taken from the third and fourth channeled phrases) is *not* imaginary. Aside from relying upon the six channeled phrases and spiritual beings from other dimensions for confirmation and evidence, the reality of its existence has also demonstrated itself clearly in practice as well as in the laboratories of science. The Reconnection is the umbrella process of reconnecting to the universe that allows for Reconnective Healing to take place. These healings and evolutionary frequencies are of a new bandwidth and are brought in via a spectrum of *light and information* that has never before been present on Earth. It is through The Reconnection that we are able to interact with these new levels of light and information, and it is through these new levels of light and information that we are able to reconnect.

By now, you're ready to acquire some idea of what this process is, where it comes from, and how it works. Welcome to something *new*. This is *different.* This is *real*—and it's somehow being entrained in *you.*

Luckily, it's not necessary to spin tall tales about the source or nature of this energy. Reconnective Healing is firmly supported by the latest theories on nuclear and quantum physics, where everything we human beings have always held to be true gets turned upside-down, time flows backward, gravity grows stronger with distance, and matter and energy break down into vibrating loops of string.

❧ ❧ ❧

❧ CHAPTER TEN ❧

Strings and Strands

*"From the multisensory point of view, insights, intuitions,
hunches, and inspirations are messages from the soul, or from
advanced intelligences that assist the soul on its evolutionary journey."*
— Gary Zukav, author of *The Seat of the Soul*

What Lies Beyond

Humans are inquisitive beings. We always want to know the "how's"
and "why's," even when the answers don't do us any good. And
often they don't. Often "how" and "why" can be two very dis-
empowering questions. Yet from the very beginning, there I was, asking
just that: "How?" "Why?" "How does this work?" "Why is it here?" "What's
going on?"

I never really received an answer that satisfied me.

I know that not everyone is so insistent upon getting answers. Some
people just don't ask a lot of questions. They read about something, and
they believe it. Their friends tell them about something else, and they believe
that. High gullibility combined with what I call "The Lemming Factor" has
people running en masse and jumping off one New Age cliff after another,
looking for answers, yet drowning in a sea of continually redirected inde-
cision.

It was only after I realized that I wasn't going to be given any more
answers—from external sources, anyway—that I came to the conclusion
that maybe it wasn't *important* for me to know. Perhaps it would even be
counterproductive. But there were clues—alluring hints that I'll share with
you now.

"What you are doing is reconnecting strands."

"What you are doing is reconnecting strings."

As mentioned previously, these were the third and fourth statements channeled to me by a number of my patients. From my own experience, I knew right away what "strands" referred to. When we use this healing energy, we're doing more than fixing some particular problem; we're literally reconnecting strands—strands of deoxyribonucleic acid: DNA. DNA is a complex molecule consisting of two strands connected in a spiraling double-helix shape, like a twisted ladder. Science teaches that every human being has these two strands in every DNA molecule in their body, and this configuration is the basis of our genetic code or blueprint. From such minute bits of matter come the structure of our bodies, our brains, even large parts of our personalities.

What science *doesn't* teach—at least not yet—is that at one time we may have had *12* strands of DNA encoding that much more information! (Yes, lock me up—I said it, and I swore I wasn't going to.) "Reconnecting strands" implies that rather than continuing to evolve forward in a near-linear fashion, the human race will benefit by simultaneously reaching back in time and bringing forward certain aspects from when we were a more complete people.

That's part of what's happening now with The Reconnection: We are reconnecting with who we once were.

♒ ♒ ♒

"What you are doing is reconnecting strands."
"What you are doing is reconnecting strings."

At first, I thought that the two phrases meant pretty much the same thing—some people used the word *strands;* other people used the word *strings*, that's all. Semantics. Then I heard about a concept from quantum physics, and I knew I'd entirely missed the point of the "strings" that the entities were referring to.

That phrase wasn't about DNA at all. It was about simultaneously occurring (parallel) planes of existence: It was about subnuclear physics. It was about describing the fundamental structure of the universe itself. It was about *string theory.*

Basically, "string theory" is a way of looking at the building blocks of matter and energy in a way that might very well clear up a dilemma that's been plaguing scientists for decades: the argument that the two main branches of physics can't both be true!

This isn't the physics we all suffered through in school. This is physics giving support and insight into life, into spirituality, into parallel planes of existence. Take a look. After all, physics is what defines the physical universe we live in. Physics is about the objects within that universe, the forces that hold it together, and the secrets that make it tick.

Physics is also about extremes. At one end of the scale, the bizarre principles of "quantum mechanics" describe and predict the behavior of the very, very small: atoms and their constituent parts. At the other extreme, Einstein's two theories of relativity deal with the vastness of the universe itself, the speed of light, and the warping of spacetime by massive bodies such as stars, galaxies, and black holes.

Apart from their abstract beauty, both theories have proven themselves to be very powerful tools. Quantum mechanics led to the development of the computer chip. Relativity gave cosmologists the tools to explain all kinds of strange activity out there in the vastness of the universe.

The problem, they say, is, if quantum physics is true, then relativity has to be false, and vice versa. When you try to apply the rules that govern one realm to the rules that govern the other, they stop working. Quantum mechanics suggests that at the subatomic level where matter and energy stop being separate entities, the universe is so chaotic and unpredictable that it's referred to as "quantum foam." On the other hand, relativity only works in a perfectly smooth, highly predictable universe.

For decades, physicists have been seeking some way to unify these two powerful theories into a single Theory of Everything. Now it looks like they might have found it—with string theory.

According to this concept, the tiniest "things" in the universe are not the subatomic particles all of us have heard about—protons, neutrons, and electrons—nor even the more arcane particles nuclear physicists routinely handle—quarks, leptons, neutrinos (which sounds like the name of a breakfast cereal, if you ask me), and so forth. It appears that the most fundamental particles in the universe aren't really particles at all. They're best described as loops of "string" that vibrate at specific frequencies. These vibrational frequencies determine the "identity" of the string, and therefore what kind of particle it will be a part of: a quark that's part of an atom that's part of a molecule of matter, or a particle that will ultimately become a photon of electromagnetic energy. It all depends on the frequency of vibration.

When viewed at that level, the "quantum foam" no longer looks so irredeemably chaotic.

Well, that might please physicists, but what about the rest of us? What does string theory mean to *us*? You've probably already jumped on it: String theory proposes that the shape and content of the entire universe is determined by *vibrational frequencies* in the heart of every single atom, every single particle. This concept corroborates the proposition that ultimately, there is no difference between matter and energy. All is one—and all is a kind of music. Sound familiar? This concept has been understood by mystics and other spiritual individuals for centuries.

But there's more. At the minute level of string theory, a realm so tiny that it can be described only through highly complex mathematics, the universe isn't the four-dimensional construction we humans are used to perceiving and living in. Humans function in a world of height, depth, width, and time. That's all we know. But that's not all there is—not by a long shot. So far, physicists working with string theory are postulating that the strings exist in anywhere from 7 to *11* different dimensions simultaneously. Eventually they'll find a 12th—some already say there are more. At the other end of the cosmic scale, scientists now have evidence that some particles not only disobey Einstein's "cosmic speed limit"—the speed of light—but greatly exceed it.

So what do these things mean to us on the human scale? For one thing, they point out how much scientists still have to learn. For another, we now know that there are other dimensions out there. Combine that with the unstable, unpredictable nature of this universe according to quantum mechanics, and you not only have scientific support for the concept of multiple dimensions, but also multiple *universes*—in this case, *parallel* universes, which is the so-called Many Worlds interpretation. Perhaps an infinite number of such universes exist, all touching ours at the level of the strings.

Taken to its logical conclusion, what this tells us is that the place where you are right now, as you read this book, exists in an infinite number of variations, all occurring at the same time. In one of these universes, you're sitting there by yourself. In another, the room is completely empty. In yet another, there's a party going on. In other words, all things are not only *possible*, they're also *probable* in some alternate universe.

Up until now, the majority of us have only been aware of the one universe we occupy. Via the new reconnective frequencies, we are now able to interact with other planes or dimensions . . . *consciously*. This is our movement from *five-sensory* human beings to what Gary Zukav calls *multisensory* human beings, or what I refer to as *transsensory, transcended sensory*— or *"transcendsory"*—human beings. With this, we are able to go beyond, or *transcend,* our basic five senses.

When the six phrases were being channeled to me, who was sending these messages? They obviously didn't originate from the person who was speaking, and clearly no one else was visible in the room. So perhaps it was someone from one of these simultaneously occurring planes of existence; someone who understood how to cross from one plane to another and introduce themselves into a room in our world.

Paying Attention

> *"The significant problems we have cannot be solved at*
> *the same level of thinking with which we created them."*
> — Albert Einstein

I used to think that people fell into one of three groups: those who don't believe in anything beyond their basic five senses, those who are open to the possibility that there might be something beyond those senses, and those who definitely believe there's something more. Yet suddenly I find myself in a fourth, smaller group: those who *know* there's something more.

What does it mean when different people who come into my office see the same entities time and again—entities who aren't named in any books or fables? They see the same angels, the same beings, the same guides, the same . . . whatever you want to call them. What does it mean when people—strangers to one another—smell the same fragrances, see the same colors and shapes, and feel the same sensations? There's no way that these manifestations could repeat themselves with such absolute accuracy unless they actually exist somewhere, and different people are picking up on them, *transcending their basic five senses.*

In other words, it seems clear that these individuals are in touch with at least one alternate universe, different from ours and yet joined to it somewhere in the quantum foam. Two universes, three universes, more universes tied to one another and to all other possible universes . . . by the vibrating strings that lie at the heart of everything.

Transsensory or *Transcend*sory

Trans means "across, on the other side, beyond." It also means "through" and "change." *Transcend* means "to pass beyond" (a human limit); "to exist above and independent of" (material experience or the universe); and "to rise above or across, to surpass." And *sensory* means "of or relating to the senses."

Transsensory, transcended sensory, or what many have nicknamed *transcendsory,* is the process or ability of reaching beyond our basic five senses. Although our interpretation and description of these experiences often rely upon familiar words representing our basic senses, the experience itself is not the same. As a healer, your patients (or clients) may say to you, "I heard a voice, yet it wasn't *exactly* a voice . . . I didn't exactly *hear* it." Or, as my patient Gary said, "It felt as if invisible hands were turning my foot, yet it didn't feel like hands at all."

"I saw them, but I didn't actually see them with my eyes," is a common observation, as is "It was the most amazing fragrance. It's funny though, I don't have a sense of smell, so I don't know how I was smelling it." We relate our experiences to our limited senses here on Earth, because this is all we've known . . . until now. All of a sudden, when we, as healers, work with someone, not only are we feeling wind in our hands when the room is still—or bubbles or sparkles or magnetic pulls and pushes—we are bringing *others* into a place where they, too, are interacting with other dimensions. Not only are *we* transitioning, but we're assisting others in *their* transition into transsensory, or transcendsory, human beings. We are taking them *across* or *beyond* their basic senses. We are shepherding them *through* and into *change.* But more than that, we're helping them to evolve *beyond their human limit,* to exist *above and independent of material experience.*

"What you are doing is reconnecting strings." Strings. What a funny little word for something that's so dramatically altering our perspective on reality.

સ્ટ્ર સ્ટ્ર સ્ટ્ર

❦ CHAPTER ELEVEN ❧

The Big Questions

*"We are members of a vast cosmic orchestra in which
each living instrument is essential to the complementary
and harmonious playing of the whole."*
— from *Kinship with All Life*, by J. Allen Boone

W hat does it mean to become "attuned" to a frequency or vibration? For that matter, what do we mean when we refer to "frequencies" and "vibrations" in the first place? You run across these terms all the time in spiritual writings, especially those by contemporary New Age authors. But you'll find that the words are rarely defined with any clarity. Do we accept on faith that they mean something concrete? For the highly left-brained, we may feel pushed to accept certain definitions on faith—and we may resent it. For the right-brained, we revel in the freedom and flow of concept. As we evolve beyond our basic five senses, we learn to communicate by concept, and accept the fact that certain concepts cannot be defined in our words. *Our language is limited by our dimension.*

We want these words, or more precisely, the things to which these words refer, to mean something concrete. Whatever they might mean to us intuitively, many of us think that for them to be useful to anyone, they must have clearly defined meanings. We have a desire to be able to share our experience with *words* here in what we think of as the "real world." So we want the meanings of these words to be just as "real."

Let's begin with what the dictionaries say. To *attune* is to "adjust to; to bring into harmony with; to bring into a harmonious or responsive relationship." To *vibrate* is "to move back and forth rapidly." In the realm of science, *energy* is "the capacity of a physical system to do work"; and *frequency* is "the number of occurrences (of whatever you're measuring) in a given period of time."

Now let's look at what these words mean to *us*.

Energy vs. Spirit

First, let me stress that I don't really care for the word *energy* in connection with this kind of healing work. For one thing, it's far too cold and mechanical a term for me. Another reason is that energy is generally thought of as being weaker with distance. The frequencies of this reconnective continuum do *not* weaken with distance. This is because healing and transformation occur by way of an information exchange—"light and information," to be precise. Although this healing may be transmitted on energy, the energetic component of this information is but one of its carriers. A simple analogy is *whispering.* Whispering utilizes far less energy than shouting, yet in the appropriate state, you receive just as much, if not more, information. Either way, what we're talking about is *not* the use of energy per se—it's about the *transfer* of information. In other words, the information transfer is not dependent upon the amount of energy carrying it. For this reason, Reconnective Healing takes you far beyond the realm of any form of energy healing.

What we're doing in Reconnective Healing is definitely more along the lines of healing through Spirit or spirituality. However, I don't care for the term *spiritual healing* either, because, although in its purest sense it is most closely aligned to what we're doing, what it's come to mean today is collection plates being passed around and people being smacked on their foreheads and falling over backward in an obligatory fashion. Therefore, this term doesn't work, either. To the best of my current understanding, what's happening is most accurately defined as a "spiritual communication/information exchange."

Beverly Rubik, Ph.D., once said that she felt a more representative term to be "Holy Information" (yet I wouldn't want the burden of carrying that cross).

So, for now, and for ease of communication and simplicity in this text, let's just use the word *energy.*

Frequencies

What about "vibration"? It's a word we use all the time, yet many of us aren't really sure what it means. Of course, we always have the simplistic dictionary definition to fall back on: A vibration is simply a repetitive movement. A guitar string vibrates when plucked; the number of times the string goes back and forth per second is the "frequency" of the vibration. To us, this registers as a specific sound. Change the frequency and you change the sound.

But the effects of vibration go far beyond what our senses are able to distinguish without help. For example, the force that makes a magnet stick to your refrigerator is the same one that enables you to see the *contents* of the refrigerator when you open its door at night: electromagnetism. The only difference between magnetism and visible light is the *frequency* of the energy's wave motion. What are colors? Different frequencies of visible light as interpreted by our brains. What are heat and cold? Different frequencies of molecular movement, again interpreted by our brains.

This continues clear down to the level of the tiniest subatomic particles. In fact, as I've already explained, physics is just coming around to confirming the long-held belief that, ultimately, everything in the universe consists of vibrations occurring at different frequencies. Change the frequency of that vibration and you change the nature of the particle that the vibration defines. When an electron vibrates, some say, the entire universe trembles.

Vibration and frequency play a role in two other terms, *resonance* and *entrainment*. Gregg Braden, in his book *Walking Between the Worlds*, defines them. *Resonance*, he explains, is . . .

> an exchange of energy between two or more systems of energy. The exchange is two-way, allowing each system to become a point of reference for the other. A common example of resonance is illustrated with two stringed instruments placed on opposite sides of the room. As the lowest string of one instrument is plucked, the same string on the second instrument will vibrate. No one touched the string; it is responding to the waves of energy that traveled across the room and found resonance with the second string.

Entrainment, he goes on to say, is . . .

an alignment of forces, or fields of energy, to allow maximum transfer of information or communication. For example, consider two elements adjacent to one another and each is vibrating. One is vibrating at a faster rate, while the other is vibrating at a slower rate. The tendency for the element of slower vibration to synchronize and match the element of faster vibration may be considered entrainment. To the degree that the match is accomplished, we say that entrainment has occurred, or the faster vibration has entrained the slower vibration.

So, what does that mean to us? It means that "to attune or entrain to a higher frequency" is to "come into harmony with a recurring movement that occurs at a high number of repetitions per second."

Think about it in terms of the *effects* of this attunement. Say you were born color blind, unable to distinguish blue from red from yellow. Then something happens to your eyes, and the color-receptive cells kick in. Can you imagine? Suddenly a whole new realm of perception comes to life for you.

In Reconnective Healing, a similar event occurs. As we attune (come into harmony) with the new frequencies of energy, we begin to feel changes inside our own body. The vibrations will register within us and become part of us. Being able to recognize these sensations is an important aspect of our learning to work with the healings, just as being able to see colors is invaluable to a painter. Please note, however, that it is *not* a requirement. Although the feedback imparted through this ability is of great benefit to the honing of our skills, there *are* blind painters and deaf musicians. Feedback systems will develop for you in their own way, out of a place of peace and stillness. The entrainment, the alignment of forces and fields, the communication of light and information, will come about and will most likely find a way to make itself known to you.

How will this attunement take place for *you*? What can you do so that your body—for that matter, your very *being*—becomes aware of the new vibrations and is able to act as a conduit for them?

Guess what? You're already in the process of undergoing these changes. The changes are occurring in you right now. For many, it's an *a priori* conclusion that this process of attunement is encoding and unfolding in you even as you read this book. For others, you most likely are, or are about to be, discovering it.

In my experience, there are three main "styles" by which people make this attunement, this shift to accommodate the new frequencies: (1) You may notice changes in yourself almost from the beginning—new sensations of warmth, a strange feeling in your head or hands when you first hear of the material I'm writing about, or see it in a store. (2) For others, your process may begin after you pick up the book and hold it, or open it and start reading. You may begin to notice things happening as you read further and further. Immersed in the material, your sensations become more and more apparent. (3) A few of you may not feel anything until a little later on—three days, three weeks, maybe longer.

Finally, there is a fourth "style"—the *manifestor*. This is a person who develops tiny blisters or experiences inexplicable bleeding, as I did at one point in my own development. If this happens, it only seems to last for a day or two, and simply means that your body is shifting to accommodate these newer and larger frequencies.

Discovering Specificity

In March of 1994, I received a strange invitation to attend an open gathering. According to the invitation, it seemed that the Archangel Michael had selected this point in time to return to Earth, and a group had decided to come together and help "ground in" his energies.

Now, I don't know about you, but I have a little difficulty believing that if the Archangel Michael wanted to visit Earth, the success of his venture would hinge upon 30 or so people "ohm-ing" him in.

Despite my reservations, I went to the meeting. At the time, I was looking everywhere for answers and was still at the point where I felt that, with all the "healers" out there, *someone* had to know *something* about this that I didn't. In fact, I was just getting past the point where I was sure that *everyone* out there knew *everything* that I didn't.

I showed up at the apartment where this event was being held and made my way through the crowd. The people were gathered around two massage tables, one person lying on each one. Some of the participants were resting their hands on the person on their table; others were holding their hands in the air above the person, "healer-style."

When in Rome . . . , I thought, and joined in.

I was there for answers— and I received several. The first came as I stood there waiting for the people on the massage tables to start having involuntary body movements and begin channeling phrases, as my patients had been doing. Instead, those on the tables just lay there as if they were meditating or taking naps, which I can't say with certainty wasn't the case.

I was disappointed. I'd hoped that the people in the room would be able to see what had become a daily occurrence in my office; I'd hoped they could provide some further understanding.

Instead, I saw less movement than in the return line at a department store the day after Christmas.

Somewhat confused by the low level of physical response exhibited by those on the tables, I asked if anyone would mind if I demonstrated what happened when I was the only one holding my hands near a person. They agreed, and moved some chairs close to one of the massage tables so they could observe and maybe offer some insight. One of them volunteered to be on the table. As the rest took their seats, I began.

The results were immediate. The muscles around the volunteer's mouth began to twitch, his fingers went into an involuntary asymmetrical bilateral movement pattern, his eyes started to rapidly dart from side to side, and he started to speak. This response didn't begin as quickly as it usually did when I was in my own environment, but within a few minutes, it was almost in full force. From the gasps in the room, I could tell that no one there had ever seen something so powerful.

Then, suddenly and uncharacteristically, the activity started to weaken. The voice stopped and the movement died down considerably. I had never seen this happen before. Finally, I raised my head and turned toward the others, about to explain how unusual this was. It was then that I saw it: The group had decided to "help out." There they sat, hands surreptitiously turned palms-up, aimed toward the person on the table. Not all of them, just some. As I watched what was occurring, I noticed that the few who had elected to change their agreement and "participate" gave others the impetus to do the same. I observed as more people joined in: With each additional entrant, the response of the volunteer lessened.

Now the idea of helping out is a wonderful one, as is the concept of group energy, yet let's remain conscious and objective here. The results weren't impressive when the group was working as a whole. Then later, in a one-on-one demonstration for the room, the results displayed themselves clearly; but following that, when the group reinserted itself into the equation, the results died back down to almost nothing. So, clearly, there was a dynamic here worth examining.

In discussion, the reason the attendees later gave for having joined in was that they thought "group energy would make the effect stronger." And while that may sound logical, it hadn't worked. But why not? Why didn't *more* energy mean *more* help?

The answer came to me clearly: *Group energy—especially a group not yet carrying the new frequencies—somehow alters or dilutes the specificity of the frequencies that actually bring about the healing*. The energies we are helping to "bring in" now are not the energies everyone else has been using. These new energies function at unique vibrational frequencies and do not benefit from having a lot of other frequencies mixed in. Whereas adding quarters to a piggy bank yields an increased sum of money, adding water to your perfectly balanced soup or your cup of coffee dilutes it— and probably not in a desirable way.

It was an important lesson on several levels. Although, as a group, we may have missed out on the possibility to share and learn something new, it allowed us to recognize that there was a specificity to these frequencies, something that set them apart from the others we've had access to on the planet up until now. Also, as I worked with many of these healers later, we discovered that, when entrained with these new energies, the group experience took on a whole new dimension . . . or, should I say, *dimensions*.

The Big Shift

How is it that suddenly there are "new" frequencies on the planet? Or, more appropriately stated, how can there be frequencies that are new to the planet if the frequencies themselves are a part of the ever-evolving universe?

As I see it, the sudden appearance of these frequencies on Earth seems to have something to do with the way time is changing. If you're paying attention at all, you've probably noticed that time seems to be moving faster. Not in the way our grandparents might say, "As you get older, the summers seem to come more quickly." This is different. Not only is time moving more quickly, but we're accomplishing much more in what appears to be the same time frame.

This might sound like a contradiction—if time were moving faster, you'd expect us to have *less* time to get things done, right? Yet the reverse is true. It's as if each unit of time has actually slowed down so that we can get more accomplished *during* it—yet overall, time appears to be moving faster. This is reminiscent of the contradictory nature of quantum physics and relativity. They can't both be true, yet at a certain level, they are.

Time, energy, mass . . . they're all interconnected. That's what relativity means. If something moves faster, its mass increases and its time frame slows down. Therefore, if time is speeding up, then the frequencies that underlie all the dimensions of our universe must also be shifting.

For evidence, just look at all the changes that occurred in the last couple of decades of the 20th century. Fifteen years ago, you might not have been interested in reading this book. Seven years ago, I wouldn't have *written* it! Look at people you've known quite well and for a long time. Have you noticed how, if you start to speak to them about spiritual matters and concepts such as "shifts," they're not only more open and receptive than you might have anticipated, but many of them admit they've been contemplating these things for quite a while in the quiet of their own minds? Closet metaphysicians. Yet just a few years back, some of these people would have looked at you more than a bit oddly for even bringing up such subjects.

In addition, look at today's medical establishment. Twenty years ago, I wouldn't have been able to make it through the front door of a hospital, even as a legitimate doctor of chiropractic. Now I'm *invited* to speak and teach at hospitals and universities—not as a chiropractor, but as a *healer.*

This shift is apparent even in the entertainment industry. Whatever its faults, Hollywood is an excellent barometer of our culture. Its success depends on its ability to determine where people's interests lie and what they want to see on the screen—and that's what they give us. During the last decade or two, there has been a definite emphasis on spiritual issues in film: movies about angels, life after death, paradigm shifts, parallel dimensions, psychic abilities . . . and, yes, *healers.* Not only that, but you can't turn on your television without seeing more of the same.

The effects of this shift are becoming clear on other levels as well. You've probably noticed that many people, consciously or otherwise, are choosing to leave the planet at this time through AIDS-related diseases, cancers, and various other modes of exit. Others, such as yourself, have elected to remain and help in the transition to the new, higher vibrations.

This transition is referred to by many names. "The Shift" and "Shift of the Ages" are two terms used by Gregg Braden. The transition was predicted by the Mayans, the Incas, the Hopi, Nostradamus, Edgar Cayce, and the Kabbalah (both Jewish and Christian). In *Walking Between the Worlds,* Braden defines this shift as . . .

both a time in Earth history as well as an experience of human consciousness. Defined by the convergence of decreasing planetary magnetics
and increasing planetary frequency upon a point in time, the Shift of the
Ages, or simply, The Shift, represents a rare opportunity of collectively
repatterning the expression of human consciousness. The Shift is the term
applied to the process of Earth accelerating through a course of evolutionary change, with the human species linked, by choice, to the electromagnetic fields of Earth, following suit through a process of cellular
change.

Now, I'm not saying that all "predictions" should necessarily be taken
as fact. I'm not one to buy into everything I hear, and I suggest that you
maintain a healthy and objective degree of skepticism as well. A lot of writings can be twisted and interpreted to say things based upon the agenda of
the interpreter.

However, when so many of these recognized sources seem to be both
saying the same things and predicting the same time frame in which this
Shift will occur, burying your head in the sand like an ostrich might not
be the most appropriate response. Predictions of this magnitude don't just
pop out of thin air. This much corroboration is evidence for the very plausible concept of a Universal Intelligence, a body of knowledge with which
some people—those who allow themselves to be sufficiently open—can
easily connect.

Edgar Cayce, Nostradamus, and others brought us this information. Now
The Shift is here. You almost have to try to *not* see it.

I'm glad I didn't read or hear about this Shift prior to noticing it on
my own. Had that been the case, I might never have been sure that I was-
n't simply imagining something as an anticipatory reaction. Recognizing
it on my own—as most of you have, or are in the process of doing now—
and only later discovering it in the writings of sages, served as verifica-
tion for me. It validated the authenticity of what we are now discovering,
what we are now recognizing, and served as the confirmation I needed to
be able to accept the reality of it and continue forward.

⁓ ⁓ ⁓

✆ CHAPTER TWELVE ✆

To Give, You Have to Receive

"[And] Moses said to Israel: 'And not with you alone do I establish this covenant . . . but with those who stand among us today before the Lord, our God, and also with those who are not here among us this day.'"
— The Old Testament

It turns out that I had to go inside to find most of my answers. From early on in my acquaintance with the healing energies, I had two concerns: one, that I couldn't predict what someone's response would be and therefore could make promises to no one; and, two, that I would have unpredictable highs and lows with respect to the energies that would last anywhere from hours to days to weeks, leaving me feeling more than a little lost and confused about my direction.

People would say, "Oh, you're feeling *down* today, so the healings aren't coming through."

And I'd explain, "No, the healings aren't coming through, and *that's* why I'm feeling down."

People did not seem to want to get this. I'm sure it went against some New Age aphorism or something . . . and I'm glad I don't know which one. Whatever the case, what I did know was that I was feeling great while the healings were occurring, but when they would go into a *low* period, I'd feel abandoned and wonder if they were ever going to return. No one had any answers for me, not any *real* answers. So I would think back to the six channeled phrases. I knew the answers were in there somewhere.

At times like these, I often found my reassurance in the first phrase: *We are here to tell you to continue doing what you are doing.* So I continued. I knew it was the right thing to do, although it wasn't as easy as it sounds. You see, it was *one* thing when it was working, but since this went against every concept of reality I'd ever had, it was *another* thing when it wasn't. No one can question the wisdom of the path you're on more penetratingly than you can. I became a bit more depressed, but I continued.

Eventually, the healings would start to gather strength again.

Still, these fluctuations in the energies coming through really bothered me. As we are all complex beings, and composed somewhat, at least on the surface, of seemingly contradictory aspects and traits, it should be clear by now that my predominant nature wasn't to sit back and watch as things ran their own course. I was—and in many ways still am—a take-charge person. In other words, I wasn't your basic *que sera, sera* kind of guy.

So imagine my surprise when I finally realized that for the healings to accelerate, I had to get out of the way and stop directing. I had to step back and let a Higher Power guide.

Who's saying this? I thought. *It can't be me.*

But it was true. Not only did the energy know where to go and what to do without the slightest instruction from me, but the more I got my attention out of the picture, the more powerful the response.

Receive, don't send.

Who said that? I demanded, searching the inner recesses of my head as if I could actually see something in there. *You've got the wrong person here for that kind of advice.* My ego was still recovering from *"Get out of the way and let a Higher Power guide."* None of this was making any sense. *How am I supposed to get a healing through to someone if I don't "send" it to them?* I wondered.

Receive, don't send.

I heard you the first time; now answer my question, I retorted.

Silence.

(Silence can really irk me sometimes.)

But as I came to find out, *Receive, don't send* was the full extent of the rule. At that point, I truly embraced the concept that I had been espousing, yet not fully understanding, all along: *I am not the healer; only God is the healer,* and for some reason, whether I'm a catalyst or a vessel, an amplifier or intensifier—pick your word—I'm invited into the room.

Receive, don't send.

How do I know this is true? Simple: I tested it. If I tried to force things, if I tried to take charge of the energy and make it do this or that, then it stopped working. But if I stepped back, took myself out of the picture, and let the energy take over, the healings returned.

I'm not the only one who tested it either. Back at the University of

Arizona, under the direction of Dr. Gary Schwartz, research was now under way. We were conducting a number of experiments intended to impart further insight into the nature and scope of this work. One of these experiments involved measuring the level of gamma radiation in an enclosed room where we were working with reconnective energy. Some of the researchers and other participants had attended my seminar that weekend. When I told them, "Remember, you're not *sending*, you're *receiving*," they didn't understand what I meant.

"How do you get a healing from here to there if you don't send it?" they asked.

I replied scientifically: "I don't know."

Typically, as the number of people and amount of activity in a given enclosed space increases, so does the level of gamma radiation. The researchers were trying to see if there was a measurable difference between the gamma radiation level in the room when we were bringing in the reconnective frequencies compared to what was present otherwise.

Later, while the researchers were analyzing the data, I got a call from them. "Well, you won't believe this one," they said. "The gamma radiation detectors registered a significant *drop* in gamma levels" in the presence of the reconnective process.

What they took that to mean—and this is a tentative hypothesis—is that while people are using reconnective energy, something is actually being *absorbed*. They're *receiving* energy, not sending it.

The True Nature of Healing

When most people think about "healing," they focus on the notion of someone suffering from an ailment or injury who "gets better." But what does it mean to "get better"? Better than what? Better than they were at some moment in their past? Better than someone else is?

"Getting better" is far too limiting a definition of healing. Thinking in that way divests us of our birthright to be in direct communion with God/Love/Universe; and therefore, to be self-sustaining, self-healing beings.

Healing, as we often tend to think of it, may well be about the alleviation of symptoms, diseases, infirmities, and other noticeable hindrances to full functioning. Healing is also the restoration of the person to spiritual wholeness. In essence, healing is this: the release or removal of a block or interference that has kept us separate from the perfection of the universe. Yet, healing is about our evolution, and also includes the evolutionary restructuring of our DNA and our reconnection to the universe on a new level.

Why "RE-connection"?

We all come into this existence with limitations. As history would have it, humanity, as a whole, was long ago disconnected from the energy lines that attune us to our own bodies; to the energy fields of those around us; to the ley lines of our planet; and from there, to the energy grid of the entire universe.

How did this separation come about? Perhaps the story of the Pleiadian conspiracy is true. Perhaps not. That, I can't say—but I *can* say that our lot in life may not have always been this one. Every culture in history—from pre-Biblical civilizations and inclusive of the ancient Greeks (whom we revere as the founders of Western civilization)—tells stories of an ancient, more perfect world. No war, no illness, no disease. Shangri-La. Atlantis.

Then came some kind of Fall—a disengagement from the forces that bound us together in love and happiness. A *separation*. Some people attribute this event to the Garden of Eden. Some cultures attribute it to a time before that.

With minor variations, this story is universal—locked in the collective unconscious of the human race, imprinted in our genes.

To varying degrees, the Reconnection phenomenon takes us back, in our intrinsic memories, to this golden age, and ties us in to our original sense of profound connection with all of life. Yet it is not simply moving back; it's moving forward to something new as well. From this wholeness comes healing. True healing. Evolutionary healing.

Despite all the talk about "going back," the truth is that the level of healing we're discussing hasn't been with us all along. At one time, our species was more fully connected and "whole"; therefore, frequencies specific to reconnecting us weren't necessary. What has been with us all along is our ability to raise our collective consciousness to the level where we can accept and accommodate frequencies of this kind. That level has finally been reached, and the universe has decided that now is the time for their presentation.

We *all* have the ability to carry this new frequency of healing. It's not a gift for a few chosen people—gurus or "holy" (by general consensus) men or women. It's a gift of this time; the intelligence and wisdom we need to guide us is already in place. As a race, we are entering a level of frequency where the untruths will not be able to entrain their vibrations, and being too dense, will simply fall away; the separations will be healed; the superstitions will be released. We are embarking on the exciting process of stepping through our fears, recognizing how so many of them come disguised as rituals of love and beauty.

Although the universe, for some reason, chose to "seed" me with this energy to begin the process of frequency enhancement, it seems that every day, more and more people are finding their place as part of this phenomenon. In so doing, we are raising our overall level of consciousness. As we leave our superstitions and outmoded beliefs behind and evolve, we prepare ourselves to assume the next mantle of power and responsibility.

Critical Mass

There will come a time—in the not-so-distant future—when you will no longer need to make a special trip to see me or anyone else to get "attuned" to this new band of frequencies. Soon you'll be sitting in a theater, on an airplane, or on a bus, and you'll simply pick up this new resonance from the person sitting next to you. It will even be passed on genetically to future generations.

I've seen the beginning of this phenomenon occur during the seminars I teach, where the individuals who attend are often spontaneously attuned to progressively higher levels of proficiency. As I evolve with it, it is passed on to the participants at the next seminar at that newer, more elevated level. And since we're all seemingly tied in to the same communication hub, those of you who have been to previous seminars discover that you automatically make these jumps as well.

This phenomenon coincides with the studies of the English scientist Rupert Sheldrake, the leading proponent of the concept of "critical mass." In a classic experiment, mice were separated into two groups. Over the span of a half-dozen generations, one group was regularly put through a complicated maze. The other group was caged nearby and only occasionally tested. The results of this experiment were significant: For the tested group, the new generation always started at the proficiency level that their predecessors had attained. More noteworthy, when the untested mice were put in the maze, they too began at the proficiency level of the mice currently being tested. This phenomenon is also referred to as the "Guru theory," or more commonly, the "Hundredth Monkey Theory."

Somehow, the Reconnection prepares us for making this transition into the shift that is occurring right now. Without having to wait for the slow and arbitrary process of multigenerational mutation and natural selection, we are continuing along our evolutionary paths toward the inevitable restructuring of our DNA.

At this moment, we are taking our first steps toward this Reconnection. We are the vanguard carrying this new wave of healing into the forefront of what will prove to be the next stage of human evolution.

⅌ ⅌ ⅌

❧ CHAPTER THIRTEEN ❧

Get Out of the Way

"The greater the emphasis upon perfection, the further it recedes."
— from *Mastering the Problems of Living*, by Haridas Chaudhur

The Healer's Role

For the sake of convenience, I sometimes refer to myself as a "healer," but the truth is, I'm not one. *I do not heal anybody.* You won't, either. If you are a healer, or wish to become one, your task is to simply *listen,* then to open yourself up to receive the energy that allows you to become the catalyst for the healing of your patient. The healing is a decision reached between the patient and the universe.

(Also, for the sake of convenience, as well as simply out of habit, I am either going to use the word *patient* when speaking of the person who is seeing you for a healing, or I may refer to that individual as *the person on your table*—meaning, most likely, some kind of massage table, although you can work on people on a sofa or bed or any other place that's convenient. When I use the term *patient*, it's not that I'm conferring the degree of *doctor* upon you—and it wouldn't necessarily help you any if I did—it's simply the word that flows the easiest for me. If you like to think of these people as *clients*, or if you have another word you prefer, please feel free to replace my term in your mind. And if you come up with a better one—let me know!)

The "listening" I'm speaking about is a state of receptivity of being. When you're listening to a sound, your eardrums are receiving vibrations of specific frequency: sound waves. When you listen "harder," what you're doing is attempting to optimize your receptivity. You might even cup your ears to increase the receptive area. When you "listen" as a healer, you bring this kind of receptive focus into your hands or whatever part of your body is acting as the focal point of the energies. It is in this receptive state that the miracle of communication attains a whole new level.

As "healers," we're becoming a link in the chain of reconnection. The healing energy comes from Source—it runs within us, and through us, emanating from us and to us. This energy is like light passing through a prism. We are the prism. We join the patient and the universe in the generation of a mutual field that consists of *love*—in the most exalted meaning of the word—and a state of unity. The patients' needs are recognized by the universe, which then supplies the circumstances that allow for the appropriate response to those needs.

How does that happen exactly? No one really knows. If pressed, I'd theorize that a patient's vibrational frequencies somehow interact with and respond to the vibrations coming in from the universe via our involvement. When the vibrations change, so do all the "higher" particles and structures that the vibrations define. Is the lower vibration entraining to the higher one? Maybe. More likely, when these frequencies (the patient's, yours, and that of the universe) interact, the waves may combine at such release points as to bring about a different frequency altogether. In other words, three frequencies may entrain to form yet a new one that wasn't present in the original set—something that's created out of their meeting—almost as if they sort their own enzymatic or catalytic event.

This seems like a reasonable explanation to me. In quantum physics, if you change the behavior of one particle, another particle in a different location will *instantaneously* react, whether inches or universes away. How is this possible? Is it because the particle is in two different places—dimensions, perhaps?—at the same time, or is it because the two particles share some instantaneous form of communication? The truth is, I don't know if that's true. I don't know what *is* true. Neither does anyone else, no matter what they say.

I don't even know why we're so honored as to be part of the total equation. I find it a little difficult to believe that God needs or requires us to perform healings. Maybe I've got no imagination, but I just can't picture God, in His or Her Infinite Wisdom, sitting around on a cloud, saying, "Gee, I'd really like Martha to have a healing . . . where is that Dr. Pearl when I need him?"

So why *are* we involved? Again, I don't know for sure, yet I feel that our role has to do with something *we* need to get from the universe, also.

In other words, it's more for *us* than for the other person. We may be a part of the other individuals' healing equations, yet we might want to remember that they then become a part of our equation as well.

For a healing to occur, everyone has a role in the experience.

Wo and the Suitcase

Lee Carroll, author of the *Kryon* books and co-author of *The Indigo Children*, is a master storyteller. If you have not yet read any of his books, I strongly suggest that you do so. With his permission, I'm going to reference selected segments of a story from Kryon Book VIII: *Passing the Marker*. The title of the story is "The Parable of Wo and the Suitcase." The interpretation of the story is mine.

In the parable, the main character, Wo, is not specifically a man or a woman. For ease of communication, the pronoun used is *he*, yet Wo, as Lee puts it, is really a "wo-man." Wo represents many of us who feel that we are ready to enter into this new Shift. And, although he considers himself a *light*worker, Wo turns out to be a *heavy* packer.

As I discuss in my seminars, the purpose of attending them is *not* to get a bunch of new "stuff" to take home and add to the bags of old "stuff" you already have "stuffed" into the backs of your closets. You know what I'm talking about—the bags that don't allow your slacks, dresses, and coats to hang fully down, and which cause everything longer than a shirt to become wrinkled on the bottom—or the bags you haven't looked at in years that you'll "eventually get around to" exploring and organizing *someday*.

Becoming a healer is about letting go of the unnecessary "stuff" that may or may *not* have served you at one time, but which definitely serves you no longer—except to keep you in a state of attachment. Attachment equals need, which equals fear. How's that for a new wrinkle in an old (long-hanging) suit?

In the parable, we join Wo as he is about to meet the Packing Angel, who is there to review what Wo has selected to take with him on his journey into the new energy. In Wo's first bag, the Packing Angel finds clothing. Lots of clothing. There's garb for all kinds of weather, but it's not organized in any certain manner, and none of it matches. Wo seems to have essentially grabbed anything and everything he could in preparation for whatever might come.

In other words, he hasn't recognized that he already possesses within himself the completion that he is seeking from things outside himself. He has amassed a mishmash of every conceivable item. These items consist of every imaginable healing tool, ritual, and theory that he can get his hands on. Each item he packed reinforces in him that he is not, by himself, enough. With each item he packed, Wo took more of the power he once owned and gave it away, vesting it conceptually—and unconsciously—in these articles.

Baggage is such a perfect analogy, as it comes in so many forms, and matching or not matching, plain or monogrammed, Louis Vuitton or American Tourister; in one form or another and in varying quantities, we each possess some. In other forms, it possesses us as well. As pointed out in the parable, "Honoring the uncertainty is the metaphor. . . . Blessed are the Human Beings who understand that the uncertainty will be taken care of as they walk the path—that the preparation they have done before is not necessary now. . . . The changes will be recognized and solved as they are presented."

I can't begin to honor all the meanings behind this parable, so let me delve into what some of it might mean for those of us who are attempting to walk a path as healers.

We no longer need to throw salt to the four corners, smudge with sage, or call in entities for protection. We no longer need to shake negative energy from our hands—as there truly is no such thing as negative energy—into bowls of salt water, nor spray ourselves down with bottles of alcohol or wear amulets. We need not use our conscious minds in an attempt to determine what is "wrong" with a person so that we know how to "treat" them. We may now allow ourselves to simply *be*—be with the person and "understand that the uncertainty will be taken care of . . . "

Our lesson is to learn to *be*. The freedom of *being* will extricate you from the oppression of *doing*. Herein lies the seed of *knowingness* that has the capacity to take you beyond all of this world's knowledge.

Now, let's peek into the next suitcase in the parable and see how much of what we've been discussing is addressed there.

This is the Suitcase of Books—spiritual books. These books represent spiritual learning and knowledge, although they clearly don't impart knowingness. These are Wo's reference books. His "stuff." Our "stuff." The books we've purchased and read (well, at least we've read the "good parts"). The books we haven't looked at yet (but will, *someday*). The notes we've taken, yet left in one of those bags of "stuff" in the closet after other seminars.

The Packing Angel explains to Wo that he won't be needing these books that he packed. Wo, of course, doesn't understand, and at the angel's request, Wo displays what he regards to be the most spiritual of his books. The angel tells him that it's obsolete. Wo can't understand why. "Would you bring a scientific notebook with you that was 150 years old?" the angel asks, "or a textbook that was more than 2,000 years old that had to do with science?"

"Of course not!" exclaims poor Wo. "Because we keep making new discoveries about how things work."

"Exactly," says the angel. "Spiritually, Earth is changing grandly and greatly. What you could not do yesterday, you *can* do today. What was the spiritual paradigm for yesterday is not the spiritual paradigm for tomorrow. What you were told as a shaman about spiritual energy that worked yesterday is not going to work tomorrow, because the energy is shifting and being refined. You are standing in the shift, and you must go with the flow of new empowerment."

Wo then challenges the angel with the phrase *the same yesterday, today, and forever.* "Isn't that a phrase about the consistency of God? How is that obsolete?"

"Indeed, it is about God," answers the angel. "But it tells you about the attributes of God, not about the Human's relationship to God. All your books are instruction sets written by Humans about how to communicate, draw closer, and move through life dealing with God. God is always the same. . . . The Human is the one who is changing, and the books are about the Human's relationship to God. Therefore, the book is obsolete."

Note that this does not mean that the book was *never* valid. A lot of things are still valid within the older, and somewhat more limited, parameters. It's just that, with the Shift, we now exist within a much larger set of parameters.

For a moment, let me illustrate with a concrete example. In the late 19th century, astronomers became frustrated because no matter how they calculated it, the planet Mercury's orbit didn't fit the mathematical predictions. These predictions, which came from the laws of motion and gravitation devised by Sir Isaac Newton centuries earlier, had worked with incredible accuracy on the orbit of every other planet (or any moving object, for that matter)—so why not Mercury?

The answer, as it turned out, was that Newton's laws and equations were only a *partial* description of motion and gravity. They worked fine for most purposes—but when objects moved very close to a massive object such as the sun, something changed. It took Albert Einstein to figure out what that change was: Relativity. Gravity, although considered one of the four basic forces of the universe, is not a "force" like electromagnetism; it's a deformation of spacetime caused by the presence of a body. The more massive the body, the greater the *relative* deformation (the "stronger" the gravity). Mercury happens to dwell in a region where the bend in spacetime is noticeable enough so that the little planet's orbit doesn't correspond to the predictions that work for more distant bodies.

Does that mean that Newtonian physics is obsolete? Not at all; spacecraft trajectories are still calculated using his "ancient" math, because it's comparatively simple and works just fine *within the proper parameters.* But step into a larger paradigm, and Newtonian math is as useless as trying to use a map of Boise to guide you through Los Angeles.

Similarly, in the healing realm, many of the techniques that have stood the test of time function just as well now as they always did—it's just that we now *have* more, and we now *are* more, so the old techniques are no longer enough. As good as they always were, within our new, expanded parameters, they are no longer appropriate—just as lanterns would not be appropriate as headlights on a car, although, for a horse and buggy, they functioned just fine. The weaknesses these techniques are subject to—requiring the removal of jewelry, the removal of leather, faith on the part of the recipient, protection rituals for both parties involved—are not present in the new frequencies.

Remember, too, why many of us who have been practicing healing techniques got involved with them in the first place. It wasn't to become a fanatical follower for the technique itself—*it was to become a healer.* The technique was simply one of your early steps in this process.

For a moment, picture yourself standing at the foot of a grand, cascading staircase. One of your goals—that of becoming a healer—awaits you at the top. Your first step is to learn a technique. You throw yourself into this technique, mastering it, maybe even becoming a teacher. *You now own this first step.* It's okay to love it, but be careful not to fall *in love* with it. Because if you do, you'll sit down, grab a blanket and pillow, move in, and make this step the center of the rest of your life. But what does that mean about the remainder of your journey up the staircase? It stops. Now is the time to bless your first steps . . . and continue upward.

Let's discuss one last "suitcase" from the parable: The Suitcase of Vitamins.

"What is in this suitcase that rattles when I pick it up?" asks the angel.

"Dear Packing Angel," Wo says, "those are my vitamins and herbs. I need them to stay healthy and balanced. . . . You know that I am sensitive to certain substances and foods. So, I need these herbs and vitamins to sustain me and keep me strong on this trip."

Wo is afraid that the angel won't permit him to bring the supplements with him. The angel says, "No, Wo, I'm not going to throw them out. But *you* will, eventually." He explains that Wo is in transition, physically as well as in other ways. "As you walk the walk and realize your potential," the angel explains, "you will slowly understand that your DNA is being changed. Your immune system is being altered and bolstered. . . . Messages and instruction sets will be delivered to your cells—and you will absolutely know that these supplements, although valuable to you now, will drop away as you gain your well-being. . . . Rather than becoming more sensitive with enlightenment, you will instead have a bolstering of your system so that nothing will be able to penetrate the light you carry. Slowly you will be able to drop any seeming dependence on the chemistry you travel with."

How many things do we cart around with us that rattle, slosh, and smell? (Don't laugh. Open some of your briefcases and bags and take a good whiff.) Realize that our bodies have the capacity to make specialized cell tissue out of a Mars Bar. I am, of course, not petitioning to elevate Mars Bars to the status of a new food group, and I'm fully aware of soil depletion, chemical treatments, and all the other things that befall our food.

Just the same, if a few of you simply put on white jackets and taped reflector lights to your posteriors, you could be mistaken for mobile pharmacies. Realize that the majority of what you're taking (and I'm not talking about prescription or doctor-recommended medications for significant health problems) *is not necessary*.

Every time we reach for an unnecessary bottle or jar, we're giving ourselves confirming feedback of our inherent frailty. We're vesting the power of our very essence in the need for external sourcing. Moreover, we may be keeping ourselves trapped in the very cycle that we realize we're ready to break out of: that of reinforcing in ourselves the illusion that we are not *enough*. Symbolically, you're becoming a bag person whose existence is dependent upon what you are able to cart around in material form.

It's time to own who we are, to know that we are the Light, and to allow the wisdom that created the body to run the body.

Ergo, Ego

We are not given an ego because we are supposed to starve it to death. We are given an ego to learn to bring it into balance, to master it. In many cases, ego represents identity: It gives it a separateness, a form that is essential to function in this plane. We have difficulty understanding the concept that we are all one. If we were the true embodiment of that concept, there wouldn't be any lessons to be experienced. The ego gives us the identity to experience the lesson in terms of a very specific viewpoint—ours. It's as if we look at the situation through a very specific window. The frame of the window is our ego. It gives us the form to look through (from a very acute perspective) that aspect of that problem. It's very much like there is a horizon, and then there is the vista of the entire universe. The ego becomes a periscope from which we see very specific aspects of that universe.

Take, for instance, a high-jumper. The high-jumper needs to go over the top bar. The bar is there so that the high-jumper can jump over it. It becomes the obstacle, and jumping over it becomes the reward.

We're given an ego. The reward comes when we are able to let it go . . . and see the bigger picture.

Remembering our proper role in the healing equation is not always easy. Patients who see dramatic results will be happy to tell anyone who will listen that *you* healed them. It's tempting to believe this. *Don't.* If we really want to trip ourselves up, all we have to do is start taking credit for the healings our patients receive. After we've taken credit for "our" first big healing, one of the worst things that could happen is that our next patient has an even more dramatic healing; and the next, another; and another soon after that. Pretty soon our sense of who we are becomes built upon an external value system. As soon as the first person comes along in this chain who doesn't perceive a healing, we feel devastated— because accepting credit for the healings automatically requires that we accept responsibility if one isn't noticed. Let me offer an analogy here that will be best understood by those who survived the '60s: *The "high" isn't worth the "crash."*

Ego also demonstrates itself in our ability to appreciate something for what it is, to recognize that our act of appreciation *is* our role in it. When we recognize that we are interacting with something that has already presented itself to us in its fullness and perfection, we will then cease wanting to *gild the lily.* Attempts to alter its perfection, to "add" to it, to "improve" upon it, will only push its manifestation further and further away—from us and from its perfection. This is representative of our sense of self-worth being predicated upon the external or *object-oriented,* instead of being internally based, or *subject-oriented.* We all know someone like this. To feel important, that person must be able to associate themselves with making a change in something—not for the intrinsic value of that change itself, but to have external evidence, hopefully acknowledged by others, of their effect upon something for the appearance of the "better." This is a form of ego I call *Spiritual One-upmanship.*

Spiritual One-upmanship shows itself in a multitude of situations, whether it's the person who tells you that moldavite is too advanced of a stone for you and that you should start with something simpler, the person who tries to heap cosmic blame on you for having the flu, or the person who can't leave perfection alone.

A wonderfully clear example of the latter is the group discussed earlier in the book—the ones who held the event intended to anchor in the energies of Archangel Michael. This group had the opportunity to witness something they had never seen before, yet their need to feel a "part" of it, combined with their inability to recognize that, by observing it, they *were* a part of it, took them "apart" *from* it. In other words, their not being able to appreciate the perfection and interaction of their roles as *witness,* brought about their joining in *for reasons of ego,* which is what ultimately pushed the manifestation of this experience away from them. This is the same thing that brought about the watering-down of Reiki. So many people tried to put their personal "stamp" on it, interjecting their own "twists," their additions, their alterations, their "improvements," that it's now a struggle to find it in its pure and original form.

Ego is also fed in seemingly altruistic ways. How about the person whose healing doesn't *last?* Now this is rare, but it does happen. They may come back to you three weeks or a month later and ask you to give them another session. This time it only lasts two weeks, or maybe it lasts six months. Then they're back again. On one level, our ego may be hurt that they didn't, on the surface, receive what the others who'd seen us received: a lasting healing. On another level, our ego may be fed by the satisfaction we receive from feeling as if we're a good person *because* we feel bad for them. And on another level, our ego may be considering pumping itself up again by just trying *one more time.*

If I may digress from the ego for one moment, I'd like to suggest that your role in this picture was to remove the interferences, or the blocks in that person's path. You did that. Twice. And you're about to go for it a third time. Once you've removed those blocks, it's *that person's responsibility* to move forward.

Sometimes we're so busy taking credit for the healings that we don't realize the inflated sense of responsibility it heaps upon us.

You and I are not the healers. We are but one part of the equation. The equation consists of one part patient, one part us, and one part God. When God within us meets God within the patient, the most amazing things transpire. This equation is sometimes referred to as "The Power of One" or "The Power of Three." Why are we involved in this equation? Is it for the other person? Probably not. As I said earlier, we're most likely involved in this equation for *us*. (For those of you having conniptions about the use of the word *God—get over it*. That's your ego, too. *God, Love, Universe, Source, Creator, the Light*—these are all words meaning the same thing and are used interchangeably throughout this book. Pick whichever term you like.)

To give yourself a broader perspective of the process, and the role that ego plays in it, you may want to take this very powerful approach to your next session: *Become one with the person, then heal yourself.*

Who Has a Healing?

Speaking of which, what does it mean when a patient fails to receive the healing that he or she expected?

There was a time when I blamed myself for what I initially perceived as *failures*. I finally had to accept that I can no more be responsible for the absence of a clear healing than for the presence of a dramatically successful one. So what does it mean when a healing session does not produce the anticipated results?

The problem lies not in the healing, but in the *expectation*. I used to say that not everyone has a healing. I no longer believe that. I now believe that everyone *does* receive a healing—albeit not necessarily the one they expected to have.

Recognizing that "healing" means reconnecting with the perfection of the universe, we realize that the universe knows what we need to receive and what we are to gain as a result of it. The thing is, what we *need* may not always correspond with what we expect or think we *want*.

Just as healers must accept their role as conduits, the patients must accept their role as recipients. The patients' job is simply to make themselves available to the healing energies, then to accept what comes along. And something *will* come along. It just might be a surprise.

Let's say a patient comes to you because of an ulcer. You facilitate a healing session, or two or three—and the ulcer remains. The patient feels frustrated, and you feel like a failure even though you know you shouldn't because, as they say, you're only human. But a few months later, you hear from the patient again. "I'm fine," he says. "The ulcer cleared up. Maybe it's because after I saw you, I stopped worrying about everything so much, and quit drinking and smoking, and I get along so much better with my wife and kids. . . ." Sometimes they'll attribute the healing to anything other than the time they spent with you. But ultimately, it really doesn't matter.

These people are so attached to the result—and it's attachment, if anything, that interferes. An attachment is a constriction, and a constriction cuts off the flow of that which you'd like to come through.

Directing the Healing

Reinforced by the medical model and society's symptom-based approach to healing, many people feel a need to determine what *they* feel is the person's problem prior to or during the healing session. This is the first step toward forgetting that we are not the ones directing the healing. Combine this with the present-day popularity of the concept of the *medical intuitive,* and we find ourselves opening up a whole new case of Purina Ego Chow.

Diagnosis is a fundamental part of the allopathic world—and a highly valuable tool when used appropriately. It's also an intricate field requiring, for most medical (and other) doctors, a lot of study. It's still guesswork, but it's *educated* guesswork. Dr. Reginald Gold once explained that, to truly understand the meaning of *diagnosis*, one may choose to break it down to its root words: *di,* from the Latin, meaning "two"; and *agnos* (as in *agnostic*), from the Greek, meaning "don't know." And there you have it: Two people who don't know—you and your doctor—so don't bother. Dr. Gold also likes to point out that it's not uncommon for medical doctors to say things such as, "If you don't have a diagnostic evaluation, I won't be responsible for what happens."

He goes on to say, "I've often wondered, does that mean that they *will* be responsible if you *do* have a diagnostic evaluation and still run into trouble?" Somehow I doubt it.

As a doctor, I can tell you that people often like to flout their "expertise" in diagnosis, using it as a springboard to maintain an externally referenced sense of self-importance. Those who aren't able to recognize this type of artificiality may be blinded by the puffery, and fall prey to desiring such a state of self-inflation for themselves that they attempt to recreate it in a pseudo-spiritual setting. This mimicking of one of the less-than-admirable sides of the medical model leads us into an object-referral-based desire to diagnose, and often leads us to adopt the label of *medical intuitive.* Medical intuition, when used to assist medical doctors or others whose profession requires diagnosis, is of understandable importance to that profession. Feigning medical intuition to impress does a disservice to those who are competent medical intuitives, and distances us from our patients and the healing process.

When working with Reconnective Healing, however, it is not only unnecessary, it may even get in your way. I am of the belief that often, the less I know about the patient, the better, because I am less likely to try to direct the session, consciously or otherwise. The less you try to direct, the more room you give the Universe to do so—and the greater the results. It's not that the universe can't work around you, it's just that there's a certain level of grace and ease that occurs when you get yourself out of the way.

Although we may not know with absolute certainty exactly what our role in these healings is all about, it's certainly not to second-guess God, or the Universal Intelligence.

How We Think

Human beings are, of course, reasoning creatures. Chimpanzees might be able to fashion tools out of sticks in order to extract lunch from a termite mound, but they don't build skyscrapers or 747s. They don't ponder string theory. And they don't open universities to pass along their knowledge to new generations.

In many situations in life, the ability to reason can be highly beneficial—yet reason, like any other tool, can be less than helpful if used improperly or inappropriately. Try using your stapler as a hammer and you'll see what I mean. (Not that I'm speaking from experience.)

The art of reason is based on the two basic rules of logic: induction and deduction. Inductive logic is the more rigid of the two: It's based upon the premise that the whole is equal to the sum of its parts. And, as Dr. Reginald Gold points out, whether it is or whether it isn't, the whole is rarely equal to just *some* of its parts . . . which is all we often have. Give that a moment's thought. Do we know more today than we did yesterday? Of course we do. Following that line of reasoning, odds are that we'll know more tomorrow than we do today, and far more in a thousand years than we will in a hundred. So if we're basing our conclusions solely upon inductive logic, I'd prefer to wait until we have a few more of the "parts."

Diagnosis is based primarily upon inductive reasoning. Human illness can be incredibly complex, particularly when you take into account the fears and expectations of both the patient and the healer. At best, we only comprehend some of the components of any illness or injury, so we make an immediate mistake if we decide that that's all there is to it. As human beings, we're more than capable of adding these things up incorrectly, thereby reaching false conclusions.

Does this mean that inductive logic is useless? Not at all. We just have to remember that it's a stapler, used for stapling. We can't use it to build a house—unless we're building a house of cards.

Deductive logic, on the other hand, is broader in scope. With deductive logic, we start by looking at the entire picture, drawing our inferences from that. For example, as we gain more and more experience in our line of work, our conclusions are likely to become more and more deductive. Our experience evolves into a form of intuition—recognizing that there's more going on than meets the eye and intuitively deducing it.

Yet even this can be misleading. With Reconnective Healing, we interact with the energies near one area of the patient's body until we're ready to move on to another area. And when are we ready to move on? *When we're bored*—when whatever it is that compelled us to work in that area no longer holds our attention!

So look for something new that catches your attention, that grabs your interest—be it a feeling in your hands, a buzzing or vibration in your ears, or a visible response in the person on the table. It's a little indicator that says, "Hey, let's work here." It's that childlike excitement of discovering something for the very first time and remaining absolutely transfixed upon it—until something else catches your attention. Are we taking this too lightly? On the contrary, this honors the process in its highest, as it keeps us "true" and in our integrity, absolutely connected and at one with the process and the person on our table. It has nothing to do with knowing if the patient needs more or less energy. If they do, they'll get it—and the less we consciously try to assist, the better off both they—and we—are.

This goes against many schools of thought, of course, which teach us to "scan" an area and try to determine where the person on the table needs more or less of something. We're taught to scan for areas of congestion, areas of too much, too little, or blocked energy. Then, relying upon our own sense of judgment, we rebalance these areas by trying to add or remove energy from that spot. Not only have we designated ourselves responsible enough to identify the areas in need, we—or our egos—have also proclaimed us capable of remedying the situation. Talk about responsibility!

How about pendulums as another form of diagnosis? Are you in a good mood when you're working with your first patient? How about your third? Did you just have an argument with your spouse on the phone? Is your hand shaking when you hold the string of the pendulum?

Medical laboratory testing is also not above reproach. Did the doctor request the appropriate tests? Were the samples handled correctly? Were the results determined accurately? More important, is the cause of the situation even something our current technology is capable of detecting? As you become more comfortable with yourself, you're able to step aside and let the healing intelligence make the determination of what's needed. I don't care if we scan the body, use a pendulum, or stand on our roofs on a windy day and pretend to be weather vanes. Whatever form of diagnosis we use, it adds one more step of separation between our patient and their healing process.

Whatever mode we use to make a determination of what we *think* is wrong with someone, we're making some kind of assumption about a particular issue, some kind of determination with our logical, educated minds, working essentially on the premise that we're more knowledgeable than the perfection of the universe. We're not. In many situations, this form of diagnosis only gets in the way because, on one level or another, it encourages our conscious mind to attempt to take charge.

In this new chapter for humankind, we've finally come to recognize and honor the intelligence of a superior healing force. We can acknowledge that this energy knows what is wrong with us, what corrections need to be made, and in what priority.

This type of healing is not about buying into the old diagnostic and directive paradigms. Our job as healers is simply to get out of the way and allow something that's all-knowing and all-seeing make the appropriate decisions. Sometimes, based on what appears to be the end result, we might not have confirmation that the decision we made was the correct one or that the outcome was beneficial to the patient. It was. We are not always gifted with seeing things from the larger perspective. Someone else does that for us. So let's not concern ourselves with what we're able to recognize or intuit. Thank God that we no longer have to. Just enter the picture, become part of the equation, and let it go.

This is the present of healing. This is the future of healing.

❧   ❧   ❧

CHAPTER FOURTEEN

Setting the Tone

"The snow goose need not bathe to make itself white.
Neither need you do anything but be yourself."
— Lao-Tse

Personal Emotions

Recognizing that you are but one part of the total healing experience does not require that you attain some Zenlike state of detachment. To the contrary, I find that there's often a heightening in the energy when my personal emotions are heightened first. Oddly enough, it matters very little whether something touches me and brings a tear, or whether I'm simply feeling very happy.

It's important to maintain a level of detachment from the situation, as an attachment to outcome is one of the few ways that this healing process can be diminished. Enjoying your own emotions allows you to maintain this level of detached presence. Happiness and other elevated states of emotion are often great contributors to a state of detachment, because that detachment is not from life itself, it's from the need to direct, the need to control. It's detachment from the other person's results. This allows you to be in the process, yet not invested in the results.

Heightened states of your own emotion allow you to remain absorbed in *your own* experience and contribute to that experience of being both the observer and the observed. This state allows the person on the table to enter into their own *samadhi,* their own oneness, where they may be in *their own* experience. Yet all is one: As the process deepens for the person on your table, you will see and feel an amazing intensity manifest. This will often take you immediately into an expanded place of awareness and observation that will then intensify the interaction for your patient once again. As this cycle progresses, you find yourself timelessly and exquisitely transfixed in this indescribable knowingness.

A Funny Thing Happened on the Way to the Healer

Let's face it, laughter is not something we normally associate with pain, disease, and ill health. Medical schools can surgically extract your sense of humor faster than a surgeon can remove your tonsils. Non-allopathic education doesn't fall too far behind in this regard, either. Visages of solemn healers and stone-faced medical faculty do little to help.

Thank goodness for Dr. Bernie Siegel, the author of *Love, Medicine & Miracles*—yet people such as he are few and far between. He presents the case that a good sense of humor promotes good health; laughter is associated with a sense of well-being, which is associated with a strong immune system and quicker recovery from illness or injury.

If you accept that Reconnective Healing is mediated through a higher or universal intelligence, and that the result will be what's most appropriate regardless of what either you or the other person consciously deem most appropriate, then what's all the consternation about? For goodness' sake, some of you look as if you need a few prunes.

Lighten up. Laughter puts people at ease. One of your initial priorities with each patient you see is to bring them out of their *dis*-ease and into a place of *ease*—physically, emotionally, mentally, spiritually, and any other way possible.

The point is: Things are funny. *Life* is funny. If you don't want to be around laughter, you don't want to be around life. As Ron Roth, the author of *Holy Spirit for Healing,* says, "Quit taking yourself so seriously. Nobody else does."

What Is Love?

When my experiences with these healings first began, no one had seen fit to send me the accompanying manual. All I knew was that I left my office on a Friday, thinking I was a chiropractor, and when I came back on the following Monday, I found out that I was something else. As I mentioned previously, I decided to look to others for answers. I picked up copies of New Age magazines from bookstores and health-food stores, flipped through the ads of those who practiced various forms of healing, and called the ones who looked the most sane in their photographs.

I set appointments to meet with these people, described what I'd been doing, and even demonstrated it. When they witnessed the responses brought about by these frequencies, I noticed that a lot of people suddenly became a bit angry. At the least, some of them developed what I'd call a *definite attitude*. Hearing their consternation, I'd ask if I'd done something to provoke it. They'd tell me: "We've been spending years learning to tune in to our hearts and work with love. You just woke up one day with this gift. You're doing everything mechanically, yet you're getting all these wonderful results that we're not." Then came the words I wasn't prepared to hear: "You've got a heart that needs to be opened."

I would think, *Oh my God, what's wrong with me? What's wrong with my heart?* As these various "technique" healers would say this, I'd go home feeling more and more dejected and would wonder exactly how I *could* open my heart. It was only when I was feeling particularly down about it one day that it dawned on me: *How could my heart really be all that closed if I was feeling this much heartache about it allegedly being closed?* It was at that point that I more clearly understood the different forms of love.

These technique healers were confusing love with the sentiment on a Hallmark card. They honestly felt that if they were able to work up a few tears during a session, it would help the person lying on the table.

Sentimental love is not the love that mediates these healings. It doesn't begin to capture the essence of the love that creates the universe. Ask anyone who's had a life-after-death experience and who's gone far enough into it to know the "love" that *is* that experience.

What these healers had been mistaking for love was *sop*. The love upon which healing is based is the love upon which life and the universe are based. It's not hormonal or "I've got to have you" love, nor is it teary-eyed "I feel for you" love. It's the all-encompassing love of creation and consciousness. It's the love that allows you to get out of your ego, get out of the way, and be both the observer and the observed, thereby allowing the patient that same gift. It is the love that allows the power that *made* the body to *heal* the body. This is when the transformation takes place. This is when the *light and information* flow. This is love.

The Hidden Fear in Our Rituals

"The most difficult part of bringing medical care to
the natives was getting them to give up their superstition."
— Dr. Albert Schweitzer

Never is fear so insidious as when it cloaks itself in the guise of love. Fear is the *only* thing standing between you and anyone, you and anything . . . including your goal of becoming a consummate healer. One of the gifts I hope you receive from this book is the ability to recognize fear in whatever form it comes, and thus transform it into love. Fear is only the absence of love, just as darkness is the absence of light. Just like when you shine a light into darkness and the light becomes the only thing present, when you bring love into a place where there had been fear, you find that fear is there no more.

Permeating the "techniques" of healing is ritual. Ritual fills a multitude of voids, including the feeling that we are not, of ourselves, enough. We then perpetuate the void by creating ritual around it, and then perpetuate the ritual by creating beauty around it . . . and it around beauty. Perpetuated in beauty, the ritual artfully turns around and perpetuates the void.

Early on, I went looking to others for answers and insights. Although I had questions for these individuals, they also had questions for me. The first question I would be asked was, "Are you protecting yourself?"

"From what?" I'd ask, looking over my shoulder.

They didn't know. They just knew that they had been told to protect themselves by someone who had been told to protect *them*selves by someone who'd been told to protect *themselves*. Customary, time-honored, age-old traditions. But *who* started this process? And *why?*

If a truism is passed on through the ages—and truth is truth is truth—then, odds are, it's still true today. But if something was false way back then—and if truth is still truth—then that something that was false remains false. It may be a lot older, but it's just as false.

Now sit down for a moment, brace yourself, and if you have a couple garlic-clove necklaces nearby, put them on, because I'm about to tell you something that might rattle a few of your false foundations: *There's no such thing as evil.* There are no entities whose purpose for existence is to hang around and play havoc with your life or hide in darkened rooms behind closet doors so they can find just the right moment to jump out and holler, "Boo!" Not only that, they don't have cousins who hang on to your shoulders and need to be pulled off of you via weekly or monthly healing sessions, or who can be warded off by expensive, gem-studded pendants. Quit flattering yourself. These are created figments and fantasies, strengthened only by your fear of them. If any of these entities ever *did* exist, they're dead now. They died laughing at all the antics you performed trying to protect yourselves from them. One died just yesterday when it found out how much money you spent on that amulet.

Let's take a look at just a few of our fear-based rituals:

- *Flowers*—to keep away ghosts

- *Shaking off your hands*—to rid yourselves of other people's negative energy picked up during healing sessions

- *Water bowls*—to catch the negative energy you shake off your hands

- *Salt*—putting it into the water to break up the negative energy once the water catches it after you shake it off your hands

- *Alcohol*—to spray your hands down with in case you don't have the bowls and the salt and the water to shake them off into

- *Candles*—burning certain colors for protection

- *Directions of movement*—turning or walking only in certain directions (right, left, clockwise, or counterclockwise, depending on your source or school of thought)

- *Directions of placement*—the patient is to lie in a certain direction (head facing north, south, east or west, depending on your source or school of thought)

- *Hands*—the right hand is the sending hand; the left hand is the receiving hand

- *Jewelry and/or leather*—remove it or it may interfere with the healing

- *Exhaling*—blowing or coughing out negative energy

- *Crossing the spine*—having to stand on the person's right if you're working on their right side; and their left, if you're working on their left side so as not to cross over their spine

- *Tissue*—to dry your tears from either laughing so hard at some of this that you blow out your candles, or from crying when you accidentally kill your flowers by placing them in the salt water you were supposed to shake your hands off into . . . and the prayers don't bring them back

We cannot come from love while we reinforce the concept of fear. As a culture, we decorate our fears with rituals, and then we fool ourselves into thinking that these rituals are expressions of love. We diminish prayer when we use it for protection, for what are we using prayer and these other rituals to protect us *from*? Nothing more than the amorphous nature of our fears—simply because we buy into the concept of evil. Yet we fail to recognize that evil is merely a specter of illusion. We spend so much time protecting ourselves from something that doesn't exist, it's no great wonder that we have so little time left over for what *does*. As our attention creates illusory embodiments of evil—which, in turn, cycles more of our attention—our belief systems become self-reinforcing. Often we simply don't realize that we go where our attention is.

Do you really think that if you wave a bouquet of flowers at a ghost, it will turn and run out of your life screaming? Maybe. But only if it has hay fever. If a ghost is hanging around, it isn't because of you. It has its own thing to handle, its own purpose for its cycle interruption.

How about shaking negative energy off of your hands and into a bowl of salt water? Are you trying to drown it? That will only work if it comes from a fresh-water universe.

The inherent problem with these rituals of protection is that when you're doing something that's designed to protect you, you're telling yourself that there's something to be afraid of—even when it comes to worrying about the direction in which a person lies, which hand to use, or something as simple as being afraid that you're doing it "wrong." So, the less you consciously recognize the fear-based derivation of the ritual, the more the effects of fear permeate. The same fear-basis applies to other ritualistic behaviors and superstitions, such as removing leather and jewelry. When you have your patient remove these items, you're telling yourself that *you're* not enough—that you and what you're bringing through is limited in nature.

Let me give you just one reason I know this to be true: When these healings first started to occur, my patients thought they were coming in to see a chiropractor—and I thought I *was* one. You couldn't have double-blinded a study better. And, of course, as chiropractic patients, they came in with their steel-toed leather work boots, heavy belts, metal leg braces, and all of their usual jewelry. I had no reason to suggest that they remove their jewelry or leather. I didn't stop to say prayers, or burn sage or incense over them, nor did I ground the energy of the room with chakra-colored crystals imported from equatorial South America. I simply watched in child-like wonder. No attachment, no constriction, no ritual, no fear. Just healings from the universe, plain and simple.

It's Not What You Do, It's Why You Do It

Saying a prayer before each session is spiritual manipulation. Just as you would know that you were being manipulated by your child or spouse if they prefaced every request throughout the day with an "I love you," you know that a prayer before each healing session is simply *you* asking for something from God, whether it's outwardly for you or for someone else. Instead of asking for something, *offer* something. You can start by offering thanks. I say a prayer of thanks every morning because I'm genuinely grateful for what I have. I then feel perfectly established in my state of thankfulness and go through the day doing what I usually do without feeling the need to ask for special protection or special dispensation.

What's the difference between a prayer of thanks and a prayer of request? For one, prayers of request lead to more prayers of request. Prayers for protection keep your attention focused on fear, leading to more prayers of protection. Sometimes it's nice to neither be hearing constant requests for favors, nor be making them. A prayer of thanks allows you to move through the day, comfortable in your relationship with the universe. I think God likes that.

What are you doing when you start calling in the presence of God and/or the archangels before each session you give? You're telling yourself that you don't really think that God is with you always, that He and the angels must have gone out for coffee and left you on your own to fend off the ghost with the sinus problems.

How do you break out of your fear patterns? First, by recognizing them. The light of recognition dispels the darkness without your having to do much more than remain conscious. How can you expedite the process? It's simple. Each time a fear comes up, walk into it. If you're afraid to do a healing session without wearing your purple shirt, consciously do not wear *any purple whatsoever* that day. If you catch yourself putting your favorite crystal in your pocket because you feel it will help you in some way, *take it out and leave it at home that day.* You can always put the crystal in your pocket or wear something purple another day, but the power you reclaim every time you lose your attachment to a fear brings you that much closer to your goal of being a healer, to shedding your illusion of separation and living in infinite oneness.

Releasing Your Ritual Dependency

Can you put flowers in the room simply because they look pretty, and burn candles because the soft light makes the room feel welcoming? Of course you can. Yet remain aware, for if one day you're selecting your candles for the symbolic meaning of their colors, you're on the precipice of reintroducing fear into your work.

As I introduced the concepts and rituals of protection into my work, the healings rapidly became less and less dramatic, although the sessions became more and more so. One day I recognized that I was no longer walking into the sessions with the same sense of joyous expectancy that I once had. I was no longer coming in carefree and childlike. I was coming in burdened with the perceived "responsibility" of the gift. I finally began to understand what people meant when they would say to me, "You must feel a great sense of responsibility." Up until this point, I hadn't. And things were better then—for me and for my patients.

One day the relationship between these rituals, the fear, and the decrease in the healings became suddenly all too apparent. I stopped all the ritual—at least all of the ritual I could recognize. I threw out the bowls of salt water, I stopped calling in the archangels and other "protectors,"and I even stopped calling for the presence of God—because I realized that God was with me all the time anyway. I did away with all of the beseeching prayers—now I simply say the happiest prayer of thanks before I leave the house in the morning—and it's all right if I forget once in a while. I simply remember to do it the next day. Nor do I shake off my hands, for I now know that it's within that interaction with the person on my table that the awesome beauty of transformation takes place—and any residue that is left with me can only be a gift.

As I released the fear-based rituals, disguised as beautifully as they were, the healings began to resume their original splendor. I realized that it was a good thing that I'd been able to experience them in their fuller potential so that I *knew* they existed. It was this knowledge—along with the sense of their loss—that gave me the impetus and intractable drive to find them again. For in doing so, I was metaphorically teaching myself to walk again, something so very complex and difficult that only those who have had to learn to walk for a second time may ever know.

What was the reason for all this in the scheme of things? Well, knowing how to walk, by and of itself, doesn't necessarily gift you with the ability to teach someone else how. You may be able to help a child learn, yet that child, with its lack of fear, would have learned anyway. But an adult who's never walked—that's another story. I was not living up to my potential. I was not fulfilling my purpose by merely standing in a room, hour after hour, day after day, facilitating healings one person at a time. I was to teach. And to teach, one must have a more conscious understanding of not only *how* to, but *how not* to as well, to guide people away from the pitfalls and on toward their goals—out of the darkness and into the light; out of our fears, and into our love.

You don't need to let go of all your fear before you are ready to experience love. You can pick up your fears in your arms and carry them into the love with you. For once you step into love, fear shows itself up for the illusion it's always been, and love is all that remains.

✇ ✇ ✇

❧ CHAPTER FIFTEEN ❧

Things to Consider

"If you push the understanding of the physiological basis of medicine far enough, you'll usually come to a point that you can no longer defend it scientifically, that you must take it on faith."
— from *Healing from the Heart*, by Mehmet Oz, M.D.

Who Is a Healer?

Who is a healer? At this point in our transition, healing is a capacity shared by all. You don't need to be firmly entrenched in a specific religious or spiritual belief. It's not a requirement that your every thought be pleasant or that you never utter a sarcastic word. You don't have to become a vegetarian. You can have that glass of wine with your meal—or that martini or margarita. In fact, most likely anything else that you like to do is fine as well. I can vouch for this from firsthand experience.

These considerations are all "worthiness" issues—and our worthiness has already been established merely by our *being*. It's wonderful to aspire to become a better person; we are here to learn and evolve. Yet the degree to which we accomplish these aims does not determine our worthiness. We have nothing we need to prove or accomplish, nothing to do to become deserving. We are that, already. We cannot aspire toward that which is already ours.

If you reach out for this reconnection, you're worthy of receiving it. Don't wait until you think your ego is in check, your life is lived totally in nonjudgment, or pepperoni pizza, for you, has become a thing of the past. That would be like waiting for the perfect time to get married or have a child. It may never come—at least not in a recognizable form.

Healing, Medicine, and the Future Health-Care System

At present, I see the strength of medicine being in two basic arenas. The first I describe as first aid or crisis care. As I said in a recent seminar, "If, heaven forbid, I were struck by an automobile, GET OUT OF THE WAY, an ambulance is coming!" And I mean it. There is no one more appropriate at that point than paramedics and medical doctors to handle bleeding and broken bones. Once I'm safely stabilized, then let's talk about chiropractic, homeopathy, nutrition, and other forms of healing. This would be the more appropriate time to give your body the chance to heal itself.

A second place where I acknowledge the desirability of the medical approach is *if nothing else has worked.* If our body hasn't been able to heal on its own, this is the point where drugs, surgery, or other extreme measures may be necessary. So often in the not-so-distant past, and far too often in the present, what we see are people rushing to their medical doctors at the first sign of an imbalance. The physicians' main approach, more often than not, is either medicating us or cutting into our body. They can't help it; that's just how they've been trained. Unfortunately, jumping to the medical approach *first* often delays important natural care, and our body has its best chance of healing itself most fully and completely the *earlier* we see someone who can help.

If we start medicating and masking our symptoms from the onset, by the time things get so bad that we have to see someone who's going to look at removing the cause and allowing our body to heal itself, our situation may well have degenerated to the point where we're no longer able to get back to being 100 percent. Also, if we take a surgical route first and it doesn't work, then by the time we get to a chiropractor, an acupuncturist, or someone else whose understanding is to remove imbalances and allow our healing to come from above, down, inside and out, we are only able to bring them the part of us we have left to work with. Obviously, 100 percent of less than 100 percent is still less than 100 percent.

If the natural approach, for some reason, doesn't work for us, by all means, medicine is the next logical route. Thank goodness it's available. It's just that sometimes we don't stop and look at the larger picture: Doesn't it make sense that if our body has the potential to heal itself, that we seek out someone who will help facilitate that process within us *before* we take a more invasive course of action?

How, then, do we see medicine and healing coming together? What I'm seeing as we enter this new millennium is a change in the consciousness of health-care professionals—the realization of many that they're not ful-filling the spirit of the dream with which they entered the profession; the dawning of their recognition that there must be something more; and their willingness to look for it.

My being invited to speak at universities and hospitals is representa-tive of the more open mind-set being adopted throughout the country. Inte-grating electives in different forms of healing including acupuncture and homeopathy was a first step. Now we're seeing the emergence of depart-ments of energy medicine springing up. I speak at chiropractic colleges and osteopathic hospitals where they're moving forward in their thinking as well. Many physicians (medical doctors, chiropractors, and osteopaths) are intro-ducing Reconnective Healing into their practices—some quietly, some not so quietly. There's an adage that science advances one funeral at a time. In many cases, this holds true for substantive progress in any arena. Thank goodness that today, the face of medicine is beginning to change. It is, how-ever, a procedure that is happening from the inside out—and it takes a lot of change happening on the inside before we finally get to glimpse it on the outside.

As the public is opening its eyes, medicine is opening its mind. It's been given little choice. So, while acceptance might take time, it *will* come.

How do I see medicine and healing coming together? Exactly the way they are.

Faith Healing

We've already established that this work greatly surpasses what is cur-rently termed *energy healing*. Also, this is *not* "faith healing." You do not have to believe in the process for it to work. My first understanding of this fact came with the very advent of these healings, when neither my patients nor I were expecting them. Later, this was reinforced by the circumstance of distance. You see, the majority of my patients fly in from around the world; therefore, very few of them arrive without a spouse or other accom-panying person. It's not uncommon for me to find myself having a pleas-ant introductory conversation with a couple, only one of whom is my new patient, and then the husband or wife will go out and wait in the reception area. The patient will suddenly pull a Jekyll-and-Hyde, glare at me, and snarl, "I just want you to know that I think this whole thing's a crock and that I wouldn't be here if [my husband or wife] didn't force me." I usually respond by saying, "Well, you already *are* here, so you might as well lie down on the table and be open to whatever may come."

It may help if your patient doesn't cross their arms over their chest and take an *I refuse to be healed* attitude, but outside of that, belief doesn't appear to play that large of a role in things. Encourage the skeptical patient to lie there with an attitude of *maybe it will work and maybe it won't.* Strangely enough, these are often the patients who receive the most dramatic healings, many times with all the bells and whistles (visual, olfactory, auditory, and tactile).

Let me tell you who, if anyone, is least likely to have the fullness of a healing experience. Believe it or not, it's the person who comes in insisting that it has to work—the person who's read every book on the subject and feels they know everything there is to know about it. If there's any one way to interfere with a healing, it's through this kind of attachment, this all-consuming and vested *need* for it to work.

Why Some People Heal

It's not the disease or infirmity that heals, it's the person. And, no matter how much I explain this in my seminars, there seems to be a continual flow of questions about whether this disease or that disease can be healed.

One of the few ways in which you can limit yourself in this process is through your belief system, or what I call your "buy-ins." If you *buy in* to the concept that a certain disease or infirmity can't be healed, you may possibly prove yourself right. I say *possibly* because the universe may override you, or offer you up the opportunity to rise above your beliefs. Just the same, it's a hindrance you need not encounter.

You'd think that anytime a person comes to you for a healing, a healing is exactly what they'd want. Yet sometimes people will surprise you.

Multiple sclerosis (MS) is a degenerative nerve disease that typically strikes young adults. It tends to progress over a period of many years, gradually robbing them of their coordination, then their mobility, and eventually almost all muscular control.

Sometime ago, a German woman came to me for a session. Hannah had MS. Her husband, Karl, brought her into the healing room in a wheelchair, which she'd required for about three years. Karl helped lift her onto the table, then went out to the waiting room.

My session with Hannah went beautifully; at the end of it, she got off the table and walked on her own two feet. No, she didn't sprint around the room—she needed to press one hand against the wall and take small, halting steps—but this was a far cry from being a helpless passenger in a wheelchair.

It's usually gratifying beyond words to bring a loved one back into the room to see such a change in their mate, but in this case, when Karl saw what had happened, he appeared somewhat less than happy about it.

Hannah was supposed to come in the next day for a second session, but instead, she didn't return for a full week. When she did return, she was back in the wheelchair.

That was unusual, to say the least, as most of the time, the healings that people experience seem to be—whether immediate or progressive—permanent. After Karl went out to the waiting room, I had a talk with Hannah. She told me that Karl had confessed to her that he'd been keeping a mistress for some time.

Our conversation soon revealed what this meant to both Hannah and Karl in terms of her receiving a healing. Rather than gaining something, they would each lose something: she, her greatest tie to her wandering husband; and he, his excuse for keeping a mistress!

As far as I was concerned, Hannah and I were here for only one reason, and I had to make sure she understood that the choice to heal was hers. "If you're not going to participate in your own healing," I said, "you might as well go home."

She got the point. After her session, she was back on her feet.

Another Reason Why Some People Heal

Resistance to a healing can take many forms, some of them so thoroughly linked to other aspects of a patient's life that you can only see them with a lot of perspective.

For example, a few years back, I spent some time in New York City. Among the people coming to see me for sessions was a group of approximately eight people suffering from rheumatoid arthritis. Not mild or even moderate rheumatoid arthritis, which you may see on occasion with someone whose knuckles are noticeably enlarged and whose fingers don't have a full range of motion—no, this group had severe, deforming, crippling rheumatoid arthritis. A lot of them had at least one hand or foot whose bone structure had become so altered that it only slightly resembled its original shape. It seemed that almost every movement caused them immense pain. What was making it even worse for them was the weather. My visit there had apparently coincided with one of those New York snowstorms, replete with icy rain, hail, and a bitter cold that chilled you from the inside out. This was weather that usually causes rheumatoid arthritics to stay inside.

Most of these people had scheduled three visits for themselves. By the end of the first visit, not one of them expressed that they were experiencing any relief. And, although I hadn't seen anyone with such extreme rheumatoid arthritis before, out of eight initial visits, I expected at least *some* of them to have felt better. As they started showing up for their second session, I was feeling a little awkward. I knew that they were bundling up and painfully making their way across town in this snowstorm, and so far they had nothing but cold, swollen joints to show for it. The second sessions yielded little more than the first ones.

At this point, my ego reared its little head. I dreaded their third visits. Some of them canceled, and I actually felt relieved. I forced myself to go through with the sessions of those who did show, but again, *not one of them* reported feeling any better or had any visibly recognizable improvements.

After that, when people with rheumatoid arthritis would call my office, I'd talk them out of scheduling appointments. I'd decided that these healings didn't work for people with that condition, and I didn't want to put them—or me—through a repeat performance of that winter in New York.

It turned out that the New York people all had one thing in common, aside from their rheumatoid arthritis: They all had silicone implants of one sort or another. So maybe the reconnective frequencies didn't work on *silicone-induced* rheumatoid arthritis.

This insight was somewhat bolstering. But only somewhat.

Later, after some discussion with my assistant, I found that these people had something else in common: They were all involved in a class-action lawsuit against the silicone manufacturer. In other words, they were invested in *not* getting well. The more information they could relay to the court regarding their lack of health and their failure to get well, the stronger their case and the higher their potential settlement—and a considerable amount of money was at stake.

Realizing what was going on with these people helped me alleviate the guilt I was feeling, as well as my anxiety over whether there was something I could have done better: *Could I have been more clear? More focused? More present?*

I remained a little insecure until one day when I was addressing a large group of physicians and nurse practitioners at Jackson Memorial Hospital in Miami. About halfway into the talk, I asked, as I usually do, if someone would like to feel these energy frequencies. All of a sudden, a nurse practitioner jumped up, and with her arm and hand extended in front of her—started coming toward me. All I could see was her hand as she came closer and closer. Large, red, swollen rheumatoid arthritic knuckles loomed larger with each step. The room around her became a blur.

"I have arthritis, and I can't move these fingers," she announced, as if it needed announcing. Not only was I being greeted by what at that point was my biggest fear in the healing world, but it was walking toward me. And it was doing so in front of a hospital and medical school assemblage. "Can you heal my hand?" she asked, adding, "I can only close these fingers so far."

"This is only a demonstration to see if you can feel it," I responded. I knew, though, that no one had heard me. They wanted to see a healing. Or they wanted to see *no* healing. At that point, they weren't going to see "a demonstration to see if you can feel it" no matter what I said.

The woman made her way up to where I was standing and held out her hand. She proceeded to demonstrate her rather limited range of motion for me and the room, giving a brief rundown of her history of orthopedic care and physical therapy and the lack of results she had received. I began the demo, and she immediately started to feel the energy—one of her fingers began to involuntarily twitch. All eyes were on the two of us as I thought to myself, *Oh, my God. Rheumatoid arthritis.*

"Okay. Let's see your hand," I said about 45 seconds later. She closed her fingers. All the way. They touched her palms for the first time in as long as she could remember. Open. Closed. Open. Closed. Her range of motion had returned. The angry redness of her joints had left, replaced by normal skin tone. Two of her knuckles remained somewhat swollen, yet the stiffness and pain were gone.

Gone, too, were my unconscious fears of working with rheumatoid arthritis patients, my *buy-in* that rheumatoid arthritis didn't respond to my work.

ஔ ஔ ஔ

There are many reasons why some people choose not to get well: *These reasons rarely have anything to do with you.*

Does this process work for rheumatoid arthritis?

It's not the disease or infirmity that heals, it's the person.

PART III

You and Reconnective Healing

"Established in Being, perform action."
— Bhagavad Gita

≈ CHAPTER SIXTEEN ≈

Easing into the Pool of Reconnective Energy

*"Busy yourself as much as possible with the study of divine things,
not to know them merely, but to do them; and when you close the
book, look round you, look within you, to see if your hand can
translate into deed something you have learned."*
— Moses of Evreux, A.D. 1240

A Note Before We Begin

This is the "how-to" section of the book. It's not as singularly important as similar sections in other books, because with Reconnective
Healing, if we "try" to do it, we're actually interfering with the
process. Confused? Don't worry. From the moment you started reading this
book (actually, from the moment you *decided* to read it), you've been "in
process" . . . in the process of "becoming." Your evolutionary process of
restructuring and becoming is so far under way by now that you couldn't
turn back even if you wanted to. The most you might be able to accomplish in that direction would be to try to ignore this evolution for a while,
but you'd soon find that ignoring it becomes progressively more difficult
until, eventually, it's impossible.

Intrigued? Me, too. This is how I ended up giving seminars and work-
shops on Reconnective Healing. When reports about the healings began to
spread, more and more individuals and educational organizations came to
me and asked if I would teach. I gave them all the same answer: "You can't
teach healing." But of course my understanding of that notion changed.

What I learned was that the channeled phrase *"What you are doing is
bringing light and information onto the planet"* refers to a lot more than
the idea of a lone person—me—standing in a room hour after hour, facilitating healings one person at a time. Somehow, when I interacted with

people, I seemed to be "igniting" a new level of receptivity designed to handle the new level of frequencies—this "light and information"—we are now being gifted with. The realization dawned on me that *an entire generation of new healers was coming into existence* out of the pool of individuals I'd been in contact with.

I hadn't a clue at the time how many people would ultimately be affected—and only the faintest concept of how profound the effect would be. All I knew then was that something vital and powerful was growing, and it became more and more evident with each person with whom I interacted. So I began to pay closer attention to what was going on within and around me as I worked with these energies.

I discovered that what I'd been saying all along was true: *You can't teach healing.*

But there was something I *could* do: bring this new light and information onto the planet—and let people learn on their own from there.

Training Wheels

Before I go any further, let me make it perfectly clear that there's one thing you will *not* learn from me: "technique." Reconnective Healing is not Healing Touch, Therapeutic Touch, or Touch for Health. It's not Reiki, Johrei, or Jin Shin. It's not Qi Gong, Mah-Jongg, or Beijing. It's not any technique you've ever encountered. *Reconnective Healing is not a technique at all.* It *transcends* technique.

I hope that you understand by now that techniques are essentially rituals intended to bring you into a particular state of being. Unfortunately, as many of you have experienced, the process of mastering a technique tends to keep you from attaining the very state that is the goal! It's like having training wheels on a bicycle: They're intended to help you learn how to ride, yet until you remove them, you'll never be able to ride proficiently—and never experience the activity to its fullest.

Reconnective Healing takes you beyond technique into a *state of being*: You *are* this healing energy, and it *is* you. You can't help but resonate with it. It emanates from you the moment you focus your attention on it—and sometimes you'll find that your attention is on it *because* it's emanating from you. This is how you begin to work with reconnective energy—by noticing it, by allowing your attention to fall onto it.

Perhaps that sounds simplistic to you, so let me ask—and answer—

a question you might already have in your mind: "How can I learn to 'notice' some kind of particular energy from a *book?*" I'll respond with the three most important words that you, as a healer, can include in your lexicon, and which I've already used repeatedly throughout this book: *I don't know.*

I don't know how people "get" their energy flow activated when I interact with them one-on-one. I don't know how people in the most distant corners of a hotel ballroom become activated when I walk through the crowd. I don't know how, when I address larger venues and can only pass through the rows closest to the stage, the people in the balconies and mezzanines start to feel the sensations that indicate the presence of these energies.

And what about telephones? I've been scheduled to appear on more than one TV show due to what the segment producer experienced while we were talking on the phone. These frequencies also seem to transfer over cassette tapes, CDs, radios, and televisions. You'll see. People will start to experience activation when they interact with *you*, too.

But strangest of all, activation is also transmitted through the *written word*—through the Internet, magazines, newspapers, and books. I'm not talking about some kind of intellectual transfer, where I describe what to expect and you think about it and it eventually happens. I'm talking about actual transmission, the energy itself passing to you through this book. How could this happen? *I don't know.* It's not as if I put on a long white robe with a gold belt and stroll through the stacks of books in the publisher's warehouse with my arms extended, waving a magic wand and shouting "Heal!" "Energize!" "Heal!" "Energize!"

One plausible explanation is that the activation is an energy carried and communicated by my word choice—not necessarily my *conscious* word choice—perhaps in conjunction with my original intent in writing the book. This certainly seems to be true of audiocassettes. I have found that, in many cases—Deepak Chopra, Lee Carroll, and Caroline Myss, to name three—the gift for conveying information is intrinsic, in large part, to their respective voices. So much is communicated on so many levels through the subtleties and waves of their voices that I listen to their tapes even though I've already read the books.

Of course, there are other authors whose voices are about as exciting as Quaaludes, and whose audiotapes should come with warnings about not driving cars or operating heavy machinery while listening—and yet something is transmitted anyway. So maybe the activation is something carried *through* the voice. In the case of books, maybe it's transmitted along with the visual images the reader receives. One way or another, it seems to be encoded in the communication. Remember, a human's physical senses are not separate from one another. They all utilize the same energy, but at different points on the bar. For example, light and sound are both (at least in one sense) vibrations—but at very different frequencies.

On the other hand, maybe the activation has nothing to do with any of our acknowledged senses, and requires none of our present-day media to carry it at all. For all we know, this communication goes on outside the boundaries of time and space while we sit here within its illusions, determined to discover a mechanism to explain it. Through our own blindness, we can end up trapped on this exercise wheel, running endlessly like hamsters.

Whatever mechanism lies behind it, the ability to activate receptivity to these energies in people whom we never interact with directly, is neither the first nor the last thing we'll discuss that I'm not able to explain. Just the same, it's a most fascinating form of conveyance that continues to occur.

Stepping Out on Your Own

This section of the book deals with a lot more than just recognizing, enhancing, and using reconnective energy. It deals with the kinds of nuts-and-bolts questions potential healers typically ask me during seminars. But before we get into any of these areas, let me reemphasize something I've already said several times: *You don't need me.* You don't *need* me to do this, you don't *need* me to do that, you don't *need* me to do the other. So why spend the time and money to go further, by listening to a tape or perhaps attending a seminar?

There are several reasons, but let's start with the main one. Why do you suppose so many people make their living as teachers, coaches, and trainers? Because as a rule, we benefit by being *taught* to do something new or unfamiliar. Instruction by someone more experienced than oneself can, in theory at least, help newcomers advance more rapidly.

But I repeat: You don't need me there beside you all the time, and you don't require specific instructions—such as diagrams telling you exactly how to hold your hands, how to move, what to avoid doing or thinking, and so forth. These things are simply additional training wheels.

As many of us remember from our childhoods, learning to ride a bike without training wheels can lead to a lot more injuries and a much steeper learning curve than learning *with* them. Continual pain and failure rarely result in competency—in fact, they tend to result in the opposite: surrender. And, although we all know that in some cases surrender is a valuable route to take, don't get into semantics with me on this issue. We're talking about *giving up* here.

When it comes to healing people, all kinds of "things"—physical and symbolic—are used as training wheels: crystals, statues, emblems, prayers, and so on. So what's wrong with using talismans, so long as they help to empower us? Because it's false empowerment. It's externally sourced power—artificial, illusory, and inauthentic. It's the result of us unconsciously attempting to vest our authentic power in external objects. Also, giving it away symbolically invalidates us just as much as it would if we were able to give away the real thing. Thank goodness we can only give away the illusion.

Visualize the following scenario. You're out of town for the day. You meet a woman, for example, and in the course of conversation, you discover that she has a young child at home who could benefit greatly from a healing session, and she requests your assistance. What do you say? "Gee. I'd really like to, but I left my portable pyramid in Toledo"? For God's sake, get a grip.

But how can you know that the time has come to shed the extra wheels, the safety nets, the crutches? Actually, the time's been right all along. You just may not have noticed it until now.

❧ ❧ ❧

✃ CHAPTER SEVENTEEN ✃

The Healer's Environment

> *"Always design a thing by considering it in its next larger context—a chair in a room, a room in a house, a house in an environment, an environment in a city plan."*
> — Eliel Saarinen, in *Time* magazine, July 2, 1956

B efore we deal with the energies themselves, I'm going to talk a little about the more temporal, practical aspects of being a healer, specifically those that support an environment conducive to healing. Many of you will choose to have a specific physical location you can call your own, one that represents *you*. Therefore, before you begin to work with and apply the energies, you'll want to deal with some of these Earthly practicalities.

The World Is Your Office

If you're like most people, when you visualize a doctor working with a sick patient, the picture that comes to mind includes a doctor in a white lab coat, a sterile-looking room, an adjustable bed, and a nurse or two bustling around in squeaky rubber shoes. There might also be some beeping machinery, an IV bag, tubes, electrodes, and some horrible food on a plastic tray . . . just for color.

Aside from when you're doing this work in a hospital setting, that type of environment has very little to do with Reconnective Healing.

The truth is, you could just walk up to people on the street and let the energy flow into and through them, and they may very well have a healing on the spot. This also applies to someone who isn't in the same physical location as you.

As your skills increase, you'll find yourself more and more comfortable working in less and less controlled surroundings. Distance healing is also an option, yet for many reasons, it may not be what you'll want to do the majority of the time.

So then, what *is* an "optimal" environment? What's in it, and what isn't?

Actually, there's not much to it: The place where you conduct a healing should simply be as pleasing as possible to both you and your patient. Following are some general things to keep in mind.

Creating a Comfort Zone

A patient immersed in reconnective energy is experiencing more than a "fix-it" job. They're permeated with light; exchanging information in a "high-level" conference with the universe. Although their awareness of the experiential aspect of their session may or may not be integral to their receiving a healing, it is a rare and valuable gift, often recognized as the experience of a lifetime. Honor this as part of your goal of optimizing their environment.

Therefore, given the option, patient comfort is a top priority. Usually the patient will lie down, preferably on some kind of massage table or along the foot of a bed. Generally it's best to place the patient on their back, mainly because this position is the most comfortable for the greatest number of people, and also the most "open"—it allows them to be the most receptive and cognizant of their experience. Personally, I prefer not to have the patient use a pillow. Not because I think the pillow will interfere with the flow of energy (a wall of *lead* couldn't interfere with this energy), but because pillows can get in the way if you feel like moving the head or other parts of the body around. But if a patient has neck or back problems, you might need to prop up the head or place a small pillow under their knees. Please note that the healings will be just as effective whether the person is on their front, back, or side, or whether they have their eyes open and are talking, or have their eyes closed and are not talking. The difference is in the experiential aspect of the session, something that often provides very valuable and life-altering insights to people.

Remember: Comfort is a number-one priority in order to keep the patient relaxed and receptive.

Your comfort is also important, because you want to maintain a certain frame of mind when joining with the healing energies, and physical strain can detract from that. Being distracted by your own discomfort is not a gift to the person who came to you for assistance. That's why I advocate that you keep your table at a comfortable height, one that doesn't encourage you to bend, stoop, or kneel. If the room is large enough, place the table or bed in a position that allows you to walk all the way around the patient. If you're working in a smaller space, as I did for the first several years, you might choose to position the table against a wall so that you have the freedom to move comfortably around the open sides of the table. This will not interfere with anything.

I found that, with great regularity, people would open their eyes mid-session, quite startled. Looking at me, they would point at or tap the wall the table was against and say, "I felt you standing over here." Somehow or other, the Light doesn't recognize what we perceive as physical or spatial limitations.

Just the same, if you want to walk around the table, you want to walk around the table.

The Effects of Lighting

As a rule, you'll want your patient to close his or her eyes to eliminate distractions and allow for relaxation. A bright light shining down on the patient's eyelids is not particularly soothing. On the other hand, insufficient light is not beneficial for you as a healer, because you'll want to use both the "feel" of the energies in the room *and* your physical sense of sight during the healing. So, a nice, neutral level of light is best if you can manage it. My preference would be gentle, incandescent up-lighting (free-standing or wall sconces) on a dimmer. My second choice would be a halogen lamp, also on a dimmer. Fluorescent overhead lighting would be a frightening choice, although acceptable if you keep the switch in the "off" position—or if the bulbs are all burnt out.

A most important aspect of lighting has to do with shadows. As you move around the patient, you want to be aware of casting shadows across their eyelids. The patient will respond to this change of light with an eye flicker that mimics one of the more common physical "registers" (involuntary

responses to the energies) indicative of a connection with the healing energies. This, in turn, can throw off your awareness of how the patient is
responding, because you'll start focusing on their false reactions.

Again, you want to honor the experiential aspect of the session. You
don't want to bring about a "false read" in or for the patient. If their eyes
twitch or they notice a moving shadow, they should be able to know that
it wasn't caused by you . . . or anything else in this plane of existence.

Scents, Fragrances, and Aromas

For the same reason, you don't want to bring Earthly scents into the
room if you can avoid them. In their transsensory state, many patients will
smell specific fragrances during their sessions, so you don't want to force
your concept of a pleasant aroma on them, overriding an olfactory experience coming from someplace *else*. Remember, they might never have the
opportunity to experience that unique smell again. So avoid lighting incense
or scented candles; or wearing perfumes, colognes, or oils— *and, yes, that
includes aromatherapy.* Also, steer clear of scented (or highly pollinated)
flowers, as well as air fresheners and strong-scented cleaning fluids.

On an even more practical note, you'll sometimes see patients who have
environmental allergies. For some of these people, the slightest residual
fragrance from incense or scented candles could trigger a response such
as their throat closing and/or breathing difficulties. They may also react to
chemicals left behind by laundry detergents (in the sheets covering your
massage table) and to cleaning fluids. Air fresheners only make the situation worse. These are situations that are not necessarily remedied
quickly—which means that you've just blown the session for all concerned.

The bottom line: It's best to leave the air as clear as possible.

Musical Distractions

When I was a practicing chiropractor, I always had music piped into
the adjustment rooms, as much for my enjoyment as for my patients'. But
now, working with these healing energies, I don't play music in the treatment room, as it tends to lead people toward a certain *created* experience.
If they're remembering the first time they heard a particular song, or thinking about how much they like it or hate it—or drifting along on the river

of thought that the tune conjures up in their minds, they're less likely to notice their *genuine* reactions to the healing process. In other words, music takes people to a certain place . . . and keeps them there.

That doesn't mean that the room has to be soundproof or dead silent. Personally, I like to have a little white noise in the room, and that's it. In case you're unfamiliar with the term, "white noise" is a form of steady, soft sound, rather like the drone of an old-fashioned fan. It's beneficial for muting the distractions outside the room. You want this white noise to be smooth and even (as opposed to the sound of "rain" or "crashing waves"), because such nature tapes often contain empty space between the sounds. Within that empty space, exterior noises become jolting.

Your Professional Attire

As a healer, you don't need to wear a white lab coat; nor do you need to wear priestly robes. No stethoscope is necessary; neither is a bracelet composed of a specific metallic compound. Just dress comfortably.

However, you *do* want to avoid wearing baggy, untucked shirts; or loose, hanging, medieval-style sleeves; or jewelry that dangles down far enough to touch the patient. Also, pay attention to clanging bracelets; loudly ticking watches; and stiff, noisy fabrics such as taffeta and corduroy. If you have very long hair (the kind that goes every-which-way, entering the room before you do and leaving 20 minutes afterward), keep it pulled back or up and out of the way. Once again, the goal is to avoid giving your patient false "signals." This is especially important with the sense of touch, because when your patients experience someone touching their arm or stroking their cheek, you want them to know that it wasn't you.

"Relative" Intensity

I suggest that the only people in the healing room be you and the patient. There are several good reasons, but the overriding one is the need for both you and the patient to remain "in process" and not to become results-oriented. It's difficult to remain detached from the outcome if you've got friends or family members of the patient watching eagerly for something momentous to happen. The presence of an "audience" can create distractions.

Please note, however, that there are certain situations when it's preferable to have someone in the room with you. For instance, it's a good idea to have a parent or guardian present when your patient is a minor. One situation that arises with certain children—and some adults, too—is that they may feel a little awkward being alone in a room with someone they've just met. The presence of a familiar face can ease their discomfort.

Aside from your desire to "do good" or "perform" for the accompanying person in the room, there is one other factor to address when you find yourself in a situation with someone's loved ones. It's what I've coined *relative intensity. Relative intensity*—better phrased, the intensity of relatives—is often characterized in the accompanying relative by rapid, intense, tiny lip-mutterings; clasped hands; sweaty upper lips; and eyes cast upward in desperation. If you're not looking directly at that person, how do you know if they're experiencing *relative intensity*? Whether or not the family member is exhibiting the classic outward signs of the syndrome, one clue would be that your patient is showing very little in the way of response. My advice for minimizing relative intensity is to keep some current magazines on hand and, explaining why, instruct the chaperone to please use them to keep their nose buried and their mind occupied. You will most likely see the physical registers begin again, and this will allow the patient to experience the full potential of the session.

Time Frames for Sessions

So here we are. Now that all the physical accoutrements of healing are prepared, you're ready to bring patients in and join them in their healing experience. But how can you know how long it will take, or how many sessions might be required for the healing to have reached its fullest expression?

The fact is, you *can't* know how long it might take for a given patient to respond to the healing energy. They might respond immediately, or they might not appear to respond at all if the healing event the universe decides they need differs from the one *they* think they need—or even the one *you* think they need.

On the other hand, I've learned that it is of little added value to keep people on the table for too long a time. From the healing standpoint, *time doesn't matter*. Some of the most dramatic healings I've seen occurred in sessions lasting less than a minute. Yet it's necessary to allot a certain amount of time for a session in order to establish and maintain a rapport with the person who's taken the time to come in and see you. If someone drives 30 minutes to see you and you only work on them for two minutes and then say, "Okay, you're done," they're likely to feel that something's a little off. So even though time is not a factor for the healings themselves, it *is* a relative factor for many people and, for some, may play a role in the benefits they allow themselves to receive.

Most people expect a session to last between 45 minutes and an hour. For others, 30 minutes is a good time span—as long as you *own* it as being appropriate in your own mind. Healing is a journey, not an endpoint. The process doesn't turn itself off when it's finished . . . because *it's never finished.* You can always evolve; you can always be better.

Sessions may be as brief or as long as you like, often continuing on their own long after the "allotted" time period is over. Predetermined session lengths offer, among other things, one real strength: They allow you to schedule your day. Believe it or not, this is important, since other people have calendars and schedules of their own and don't want to wait indeterminable periods of time until your pendulum deigns that a session is complete.

How many sessions are required? As many as it takes for the person to accept the healing. Just as no two snowflakes are alike, neither are any two healing sessions. For that matter, neither are any two people. Bearing this in mind, some people may select *several* sessions; others, one. I do tend to feel that if no clearly recognizable change has occurred by the end of the third visit, this may not be the most appropriate path for the patient to attain their consciously intended results. This is not "therapy," and coming in on an ongoing basis is neither required nor desirable.

Most of my patients have flown in to see me. They've had to make plans in advance, taking into consideration time off from work, round-trip airfares, and hotel accommodations. So, naturally, they wanted to have some idea of how long they would be in L.A. and how many visits would be required. Many wanted to keep their time away from their work and family to a minimum. For these reasons, I found that I preferred to schedule sessions on consecutive or alternating days. I didn't want to keep my patients away from home any longer than necessary, and I didn't want them to have to leave before they felt complete.

When asked how long it would all take, "three" would often come out of my mouth. "Stay long enough to have three sessions. You can decide from visit to visit whether you'd like to keep your second and third sessions, but at least you'll have the time reserved should you decide." Besides, people repeatedly told me that, although each visit was unique, there was something particularly special about visit number three.

I'm not telling you that three visits is the required number. One visit—perhaps even *part* of one visit—may be plenty. If the people who come to see you are local, and your schedule permits, you may choose to set appointments as you go along.

Be aware of those individuals who may be developing a sense of dependency on you. Patients don't need to come in for regular weekly visits, or see you on any kind of "ongoing" basis. Some people come to doctors and healers simply to get a little attention, and that's not what Reconnective Healing is about.

Also, this is not about processing. People on your table do not need to lie there crying and reliving old, painful experiences. This keeps them mired in the past instead of allowing them to move forward. The universe recreates itself around our picture of reality. If we continue to replay our old tapes, we tend to reproduce them as well. The concept of "no pain, no gain" is definitely no longer applicable.

Two things allow themselves to function within our illusory boundaries of time: our decision to accept the healing, and the immediacy and fullness of its demonstration. If someone is crying and processing on your table, you may elect to let them know that this does not have to be a part of their experience. If a *number* of people are lying there crying and processing, realize that it is *you* who are having trouble letting go of this belief—and the people who come to see you are merely picking up on it. Let's do them—and ourselves—a favor, and release this old concept. It is only holding us back. The healings that you witness will take place in an instant—with, and most likely by—the force of grace.

Current Medication

Patients are going to ask you, "Should I stop taking my medications before I come in for a healing session?" Tempting as it may be, I suggest that you refrain from giving them advice in this area for several reasons. An important one is: Unless you're the patient's medical doctor, you don't want to be playing God with their current medical treatment—that's what the M.D. went to school for. There can be severe ramifications for this—physically, emotionally, ethically, and even legally. Don't set yourself up for that.

But there's another reason for not meddling with a patient's existing medical treatment: I recall one patient looking peculiarly uncomfortable during his session. I asked what was wrong and found that he had decided to stop taking his medications. In response, he developed a disconcerting itching problem and was unable to lie still and fully experience the visit.

Why throw a new variable into the situation? If a patient has achieved a state of balance with their medications (as is often the case with those who have been taking certain drugs over an extended period of time), suddenly removing one or more of them can yield unanticipated, and sometimes unpleasant, results.

🔊 🔊 🔊

❧ CHAPTER EIGHTEEN ❧

Igniting the Healer in You

*"The greatest revolution in our generation is the discovery
that human beings, by changing the inner attitudes of their minds,
can change the outer aspects of their lives."*
— William James

Before you can begin applying reconnective energy, it's best to learn to recognize it. It's ready to meet you now—but like a stranger waiting for you at the airport, it helps if this energy is identifiable. How can we learn to recognize something we've never felt before? Are descriptions in a book really enough?

One of the most striking things you'll discover when you start interacting with this energy is that, unlike some of the older technique-based healing approaches, this process gives us very clear signals that it's there and that we're involved with it. In that regard, it's not "subtle energy"—*it's anything but subtle*—nor is it something you have to spend a lifetime cultivating a sensitivity to. Reconnective Healing isn't just something *we* feel, or something the *patient* feels—it's something we can actually see at work.

Let me reemphasize: Your connection with this energy has been developing the entire time you've been reading this book.

Now it's time to take it one step further.

Activating the Hands

When I teach seminars, the first "hands-on" part of the session is almost literally that: I "activate" your hands. By "activate," I mean that I help allow for an opening for you to receive this healing energy and act as a conduit for it to pass from the universe to you. This step is the catalyst for a process that starts you on your journey into the shift, enabling you to carry and accommodate these new frequencies.

Because our hands are so consciously receptive, that's the part of the body I use as a sort of "lightning rod" for bringing the energy through. I begin by asking each participant to hold out one hand in "normal anatomic position." This is medical terminology for the position your hands automatically assume when you're not conscious of them. To find normal anatomic position, simply allow your arms to fall to your sides, letting your hands hang loosely. Shake them a little just to release any residual tension. Now, without moving them, look down and notice the position they've fallen into: fingers gently curved, most likely not touching one another. This is normal anatomic position. It's the position, give or take, that you'll want your hands to remain in while you work. This is a position of ease. If we want to assist people with, among other issues, "dis-ease," then we want to begin from a position of "ease" ourselves. This concept of ease permeates every aspect of Reconnective Healing. Our hands are held in a position of ease, we keep our bodies in a place of ease, our minds and thought processes remain in a state of ease, and, as much as possible, the patient is at ease.

To activate your hands, I position my own hands, which I also maintain in normal anatomic position, about a foot apart, with one of the recipient's hands in between.

And then it begins. I simply "feel for it, find it, and stretch it," allowing the energy that I've already brought up in my own hands to expand and flow back and forth between my palms, often enveloping not just my hands, but also my forearms—and therefore not only *around,* but *through* yours. This energy then travels throughout the rest of your body, often making itself known in certain places such as your head or heart. This process activates your latent receptivity to accessing these new healing frequencies. There is an entrainment of resonance, one person to the other, somewhat reminiscent of the way clocks with pendulums will entrain to one another when they are in the same room.

An activation serves another purpose as well: It demonstrates the reality of the energy to the participants, because they can *feel* it in their hands. These frequencies are highly and unmistakably palpable. The exact sensations people experience may differ from individual to individual and even from one hand to the other, yet there is a distinct thread of continuity that becomes incontrovertibly apparent as you hear more and more of the participants' experiences. It's common to hear reports of everything from tingling, throbbing, cold, heat, pushing, and pulling, to a feeling like wind coming through one's hands.

This variability is important to remember, because we tend to throw judgment onto everything we experience based on the stories we've heard. For example, in Western culture, the color white is generally perceived as representing "good"; black as representing "bad." But in other cultures, *white* is the color of death.

We think of a healer's hands as being warm, and consider cold to not be indicative of healing, but rather to indicate sickness or death. In many Asian schools of healing, heat represents healing from the earth, and cold represents healing from the heavens. Neither is better nor worse than the other. We can't live in such limiting and defining boxes and expect to have an appropriate perspective on the larger picture. It's this variability—and its determination by a Higher Power—that allows for what's most appropriate to come through. This process is self-regulating, self-determining, self-adjusting, and always perfectly responsive.

Reconnective Healing provides a perspective on these beliefs that points out the futility of trying to attribute specific meaning to them. The sensations that come to you and your patients are specifically a part of your process, representative of what you—and they—need and are receiving.

That's fine, but what does it *mean* when people feel—actually *feel*—these unexpected sensations in their hands? It's as if we were given certain kinds of *receptor cells* with appropriate DNA encodements to "switch on" at their time of our interaction with these frequencies. And now is that time. When our hands—or any part of us—become activated, these receptors come to life—and once that happens, the receptivity is there; it's an element of who we are from this point forward.

This is important for you to understand because, after you've felt the energy once, you can find it again simply by placing your attention on it. You've begun the shift into carrying and accommodating these frequencies.

Responding to the Energy

Another thing about the sensations that you feel when your hands are activated is that they vary in intensity as well as character. Some people gasp or laugh out loud at the magnitude of energy they feel in their hands;

a few frown and strain, desperate to say, "I feel something!" And a very few people are, at first or until they work with it, oblivious to the difference between this and whatever "technique" they had been used to. Oftentimes, this is because they default onto the familiar, that first step on the cascading staircase they found and fell in love with so long ago. Soon the frequencies of Reconnective Healing make themselves unmistakably known, and most of the time these people report that they can no longer find the energies of their previous technique.

It's not that those energies were "lost." It's more as if they were washed over by, and incorporated into, the reconnective frequencies, much as an ocean wave can wash over a small puddle on the shore. Although you may never find that specific puddle again, it isn't lost; it has simply become part of the larger whole. In other words, you've begun to ascend the staircase.

If you touch a wall with your hand, you'll know it immediately. If someone else touches it, they'll know it immediately, too, and will describe the sensation very much the way you would. Obviously, neither of these qualities is necessarily true of the energies people sense when their bodies are activated. So a skeptic might predictably say, "That's because this 'activation' is imaginary. The strength and nature of the sensations people feel is based on the power of their imaginations, not on the power of some actual force. In other words, it doesn't exist."

That's an understandable assumption, yet in today's world of discoveries, we've found out otherwise.

Among the experiments we conducted at the University of Arizona was one where we placed a group of students in a completely sealed room. The walls and ceiling were black, there were heavy curtains over the windows, and the doors were all locked. We wanted no uncontrolled exterior influences to enter.

The design of the experiment was this: Three people would rotate randomly among three different roles—The Receiver, the Sender, and the Transcriber. The Receiver was wearing a thick, fur-lined blindfold. The Sender's job was to direct energy toward the Receiver; the Transcriber's job was to time each session and note the results. In addition, several video cameras were positioned to record everything, including all body movements and voices.

The goal of the study was simple: to determine if the Receiver, cut off from virtually all physical stimuli, could detect when and where energy was being directed. In practice, the Receiver would hold his hands in one of two predetermined positions—sometimes in an active motion, sometimes at rest. The positions and their passive or active components were randomly selected. The Sender would direct energy toward the Receiver's right or left hand, and the Receiver would verbally indicate in which hand the energy had been detected. The Transcriber selected a randomized preprinted card, and holding it up for view by the Sender, read the selected hand position to the Receiver. Only the Sender and Transcriber could read which hand the energy was to be directed toward.

There was, of course, a 50/50 chance of the Receiver simply guessing correctly—the same odds as tossing a coin.

We ran the experiment for five consecutive days. On day one, the average number of "hits" was approximately 65 percent, well above the 50 percent average that would represent a "random" result. On day two, the percentage increased. On day three, it increased further still. On day four, probably because everyone was stressed from being locked up in a lab for ten hours a day, the accuracy took a dip. But on the final day of the experiment, day five, the accuracy level was not only back up, it extended all the way into the low 90s—and for some people, peaked at about 96 percent.

That result is so far beyond the amount deemed "statistically significant" that there's no point talking about the *chances* of this energy being imaginary. The elegance and simplicity of this study shows the development of a learning curve in detecting the reconnective energies—a good, clear learning curve. And, of course, you can only develop a learning curve for something . . . if that *something* exists.

Hands-Free

As we've already discussed, with Reconnective Healing, people tend to focus on their hands. Well, why not? But the truth is you don't *need* to use your hands with these energies. You could have them surgically removed and the healing energy wouldn't be affected at all—although I'm not willing to be the model for that study. I've participated in healings where I used nothing but my eyes; I've even participated in healings where the patient was several thousand miles away.

Still, I prefer to use my hands, and most of you probably will, too. The truth is: I'm not 100 percent interested in doing lengthy sessions using only my eyes. With so little movement on my part, there's not a great deal of sensed interaction with the energies, so the sessions become less interesting than they could be. For now, this is what *I* do and what I recommend that *you* do. Why? Because even though this energy is invisible, we, the people using it, are physical creatures. Using your hands helps you focus your attention. It keeps you in the now, it keeps you in the present . . . it keeps you in the process.

The Group Process

Despite the fact that by activating yourself through reading this book, you may not *need* any help in further acquiring or developing your connection with the Reconnective Healing frequencies, I nevertheless recommend that, if at all possible, you attend a Reconnective Healing seminar where your hands can be activated in person. The true simplicity with which these frequencies can be mastered is rarely so apparent as during these weekends.

By reading this book, the levels to which these frequencies unfold within you may catch up to the levels of those who've attended the seminars, yet it may also take longer. One reason may be the degree of intensity brought forth through live interaction. Another reason is that we can be our own worst enemies. In endeavors of simplicity such as this, we are often clouded by the belief that something possessing the power and magnitude of these frequencies must require more procedure or complexity than we've either been given or were able to comprehend and implement from reading these pages. And, while books are often a source of knowledge, seeing and experiencing something firsthand takes us *beyond* knowledge.

In your seeing comes your "knowingness"; in your "knowingness" lies your mastery. There's a lot to be said for spending a weekend immersed in these energies. There's a lot to be said for the direct supervision, for the immediate feedback to your questions, and for your evolution as you find yourself able to carry and accommodate higher and higher levels of the frequencies. Seeing and meeting others as they go through these experiences with you lends additional substance. Being part of such a vast and immediate shift—seeing not only yourself but also others move toward mastery with such ease—offers a degree of confidence and understanding beyond what can be imparted through the written word.

Seminars and books offer complementary value. Whereas the seminars allow you the personal interaction, intensity, and dynamism of free-flowing exchange, books present you with material that is often more thought out and concise—appealing to, and interacting with, a different aspect of your consciousness. You read and absorb books at a different pace—*your pace*—and the information is encoded and incorporated into your essence differently, not to mention being readily available for instant reference.

What you can't get from these pages, though, is the priceless interaction that is afforded by the questions, uncertainty, skepticism, and surprise seen in others. The process of discovery is amazingly different in every seminar, yet in each case, the unpredictability and bare honesty of the shared emotions contributes to the evolution of each group as a whole.

Everyone comes in at the same level no matter what their experience or educational background—and believe you me, it's vast. The groups are approximately 50 percent male, 50 percent female. You'll find Reiki Master Teachers and massage therapists, housewives and students, doctors and nurses, clergy members and construction workers, scientists and school teachers, computer analysts and government officials, plumbers and electricians, bankers and lawyers. And, in most seminars, you'll also find the person who didn't want to come sitting next to the person who brought them anyway.

The constant diversity in the room is your assurance that over the course of a weekend, the nature of this work as it applies to nearly every aspect of life is addressed. Those locked into their left brains at the beginning of the seminar have often evolved so far beyond such limitations by the end that you are left to wonder if only a day or two have really passed. And when you notice that the construction worker is functioning with the same confidence and integrity as the Reiki Master Teacher—right there in that moment—you can't help but realize the simple beauty of this gift.

These seminars are not about some prophet or guru standing behind a podium lecturing to a group of students sitting in passive attention. They are about us creating atmospheres of interactive participation that promote exploration and learning; they are about sharing the group experience. What happens when a group works together with these energies is that everyone's levels rise at an astounding speed. It's as if there's some kind of a field that connects everyone more intensely in a group setting, expediting our new evolution exponentially. We're all changing in every second—and that's a lot to say about spending a weekend immersed in the energies . . . together.

Reach for the Energies

Let's say you've decided to try finding and feeling these energies on your own. What do you do? Stand before a full-length mirror, allowing your hands to assume normal anatomic position, nicely relaxed. Next, look in the mirror as you gently raise your forearms from your elbows, bringing your palms facing one another, one upward and the other downward, with approximately six inches in between. Be sure that your hands are not touching one another. At this point, they should naturally rotate so that the fingers of your right hand are pointing toward the ten o'clock position, while the fingers of your left hand are pointing toward two o'clock.

Now place your attention on the palms of your hands and wait for a sensation to arrive. It may feel like a pressure, a tingling, or a density change in the air. It may feel like a breeze. It may also have components of temperature change, heaviness, buoyancy, expansion, electricity, and/or magnetic pushing or pulling. Don't obsess about visualizing it flowing in any given direction, or it being any specific color. Simply place your attention on your hands and wait for it to arrive.

Usually the sensation will center itself in your palm. Sometimes it will be strong and unmistakable; other times, or for certain people, it might feel weak in the beginning. You may experience other sensory reactions as well— seeing, hearing, or smelling things that don't appear to be originating in the room, or even on the planet. A few people may experience nothing at all—at least not at first. . . .

One of the benefits of undertaking research is that we were able to explore, from a more scientific perspective, whether some of these sensations were really a feeling of energy flow, or whether they were just some kind of nerve or vascular response brought about by the position of the arm or hand.

Preliminary testing was conducted on volunteers who held their hands high, low, sideways, supported on tabletops and chair arms (padded and unpadded), and floating free in the air for varying lengths of time. The result was that vascularity (physically induced alterations of the flow of blood or other fluids) was ruled out as a cause of this sensation. What's interesting about this is that physiologic change comes about very rapidly for both the facilitator and the test subject, often showing itself via visible skin changes and involuntary muscle movement in as little as 15 to 45 seconds into the session—and virtually instantaneously, once one learns to recognize it.

Having said all that, let me make two important points: The first is, as stated earlier, *this is not a technique.* Although I may be describing to you one way to find an initial position of ease (normal anatomic position) to allow your hands to feel the energies, once you've found it, you may find it in whatever way you choose.

The second point is: *Don't force it.* Allow the sensation to arrive on its own. It will. This is not about trying, pushing, or sending. Simply place your attention into the palms of your hands and wait until the sensation arrives. Let go of your mind, ego, and expectations, and merely allow what's going to happen, happen.

Is It Working?

Let me take the point about "stepping aside" a bit further: You don't necessarily have to *feel* a response at all to be having a response! This is important to understand if you intend to work with this energy. Now is a good time to let go of judging and assessing; at this point, it will only get in your way.

What I mean by judging and assessing is placing value on the sensation, or making it right or wrong. I'm not talking about letting go of your power of discrimination, which allows you to take note of the various sensations you're experiencing. This maintains your interest and keeps you in the moment. Judging them, however, has the potential to interfere with their flow. Whatever form the sensations take—that's the appropriate form for that interaction. Keep in mind that the reconnective frequencies are self-adjusting and self-regulating, and are guided by the Higher Intelligence of the universe.

Healings come about through unity and oneness. Judgment in the way of right, wrong, good, and bad brings about separation. One of the best ways to enhance your ability as a healer is to remain in a state of nonjudgment. A first step in this direction would be to see if you can go five minutes without judgment. Don't initially attempt one day, or even one hour. This will most likely set you up for failure, as our patterns of judgment are so deeply ingrained in us. Once you've mastered five-minute periods, extend to ten, then fifteen, and then twenty. It's not so much whether you can stay completely out of judgment as it is that you develop an awareness of its presence in your life. I'm not suggesting that we can or do throw judgment out the window. Just as we are given ego for a purpose, we are given judgment for a reason as well.

❦ CHAPTER NINETEEN ❦

Finding the Energy

"The only way to know a person or anything else in the
so-called external world, is through feeling your body.
The whole cosmos is experienced as sensations in the body."
— from *Living This Moment, Sutras for Instant Enlightenment*

Demystifying the Process

Once you have some idea of how the energy resonates with you personally, it's time to start playing with it. "Playing" is an important concept in Reconnective Healing. It's not about being frivolous or silly; it's about developing a sense of relaxation and wonder while you're working with these frequencies. Remember, all you're doing is interacting with the energies for the purpose of allowing a change in the other person. You're not trying to aim it, focus it, smooth it, or change its color or vibrational frequency. You're just playing with it and enjoying its evolution.

This concept can be amazingly difficult for some people to comprehend. It seems almost too simple, too uncomplicated, too childlike. Yet, to truly master these energies, remaining childlike is essential.

Reconnective Healing is neither a technique nor a collection of techniques. It has little to do with rules or procedures. It's a new state of being. It becomes *you*. You become *it*. And you are forever changed. Period.

For those of you who have studied various techniques, you may very well have been exposed to some of the initial exercises I'm about to take you through. Although some of the methods for getting in touch with these sensations may be old hat to you, don't be confused: *You are now doing it with something else.* You are now bringing through something new and different. This will become all too apparent to you very shortly.

Focusing Attention

Hold your hands in normal anatomic position, palm-facing-palm in the manner we described earlier, with a foot or so of space between them. Now gently feel the energy in either palm, or in both. Wait for it and allow it to arrive. If you're feeling energy in only one of your two palms, then slightly open your hands so that both palms are in view. Look into the palm where you're able to feel the energy. Take note of what that energy feels like, and now look into the other palm. Simply wait for that sensation to arrive there. It will usually do so within a matter of 10 to 15 seconds. Once it arrives, bring your eyes back into your other hand and wait for the sensation to return. Repeat the process slowly, and then at varying speeds. For some of you, the sensation will be moving back and forth from hand to hand as you do this. For others, the sensation will remain in both hands and continue to grow in intensity.

The Ping-Pong Ball

Now that you've mastered this process through your attention, we're going to give some shape and substance to the sensation. Visualize and feel the energies in the shape of a Ping-Pong ball. Imagine this ball in one of your hands, then gently give it a little "flip." As you do so, visualize the trajectory or path that the ball would follow as it arcs to the other hand. Place your attention in the receiving hand, and again wait for the feeling of the ball landing there. Once it lands, give it a little flip and wait for it to arrive again in the opposite hand. Sometimes in the beginning, it takes the ball a little longer to travel and arrive from hand to hand. It's simply a matter of your getting comfortable with the process and becoming familiar with the sensation.

The Slinky

This is a variation of the Ping-Pong ball process. You can imagine the energy as a kind of etheric Slinky. If you're not familiar with the Slinky, it's a simple toy consisting of a flat spring coiled into a kind of loose cylinder. On second thought, if you're not familiar with the Slinky, you're most likely a space alien and therefore don't need to be reading this section.

If you grasp one end of the Slinky and toss the rest of the cylinder away from you, it will uncoil to an amazing length, then snakily return. You can also "dump" the coils from one hand to another, then back again, back and forth, setting up a rhythm that makes the Slinky pulse from hand to hand.

Another image you can use to help you get a feel for this energy is that of the Slinky in the upturned palm of one hand. Send it up and visualize it forming an arc as it leaves one hand passing into the other. Feel the weight leaving your hand. Now feel that same weight coming down into the other hand in incremental units until the entire Slinky lands. Reverse the process and play with it at varying speeds.

In the beginning, use your eyes to track the flow of the energy from one hand to the other. Eventually, using your eyes will no longer be necessary.

Feel for It, Find It, Stretch It

When you feel the energy (or even if you don't), imagine that there's some sort of an ethereal attachment connecting the insides of your palms, like a soft taffy you can pull. Without changing the position of your hands— in other words, allowing them to remain in normal anatomic position— feel the energy move and stretch. You may want to move your hands slowly in small circles before you begin the stretch to help you become familiar with this new sensation. This process also serves to help you locate the positional relationship between your hands, which allows you to feel the sensation most distinctly. While maintaining the sensation in your hands, I want you to slowly draw them farther apart, bringing the sensation with you all the while—because each end of this "ethereal taffy" is attached to the palms of your hands: one end to one palm, one end to the other. As you stretch the taffy by slowly pulling your hands farther apart, you can feel the ethereality of the pull. If the sensation lessens at any point, bring your hands back together somewhat, and repeat the small circle process once again until the sensation returns. Then resume stretching.

There's no need to move quickly when you're first learning to experience this process. Take your time. Play with it. Later, when you're working with patients, you'll want to remember that you have only one responsibility: to clearly *receive* and *feel*. That's all you're doing now.

When you reach this point, the next step is to begin to work with something or someone between your hands. Start off simply, with someone's hand in the space between yours, and then repeat the above exercise. After that, you may expand on it by placing your hands on either side of someone's body, and again, repeat the above exercise. Remember, for the sake of this process, that person's hand or body *does not exist*. You are simply allowing the energy to pass between *your* hands; you are not trying to send it through theirs.

The Floating Exercise

The next exercise you will want to do is called *Floating*. Imagine that the room in which you're standing is filled with water up to the lower part of your chest. Starting with your hands and arms in normal anatomic position, allow them to float up to the water's surface. Feel their buoyancy as the water supports them. Also, allow yourself to feel the surface tension of the water lightly supporting the palms of your hands. While there, notice the various sensations you experience. When you're working with a patient on your table, this is one of the ways in which you'll be able to establish a connection with their energetic field. Doing this correctly will, in most people, initiate demonstration of their registers (involuntary physical responses, which are often visible).

If You Can't Find It, You're Trying Too Hard

In the beginning, there may be times when you're not always sure that the energy is present. The only way it won't come through is if you're afraid it won't—or if you're trying too hard. Once activated, it *is* coming through you. It's already there. You'll never lose it. However, to help you find it during these moments of uncertainty, gently bring your eyes up, looking off to one side or the other. This eye position is one you will often see someone take when listening intently on the phone. It accesses the part of your brain that listens and interprets—not only with your ears, but with your very essence. Don't try to *send* the energy; this isn't about forcing or pushing. This is about *receiving*. This is about "listening" for another sensation. This is about "listening" with a different sense.

If you wait to receive and feel the energy, the other person will usually feel it, too. They'll be able to confirm the sensation. That's one way you'll know that it's still there; you've got it. In time, the sensation will become as familiar to you as the sensation of water or wind on your skin.

Although our focus of attention is on "receiving," these exercises contain an element of "sending" as well. Remember that their design is to help you tune your perceptions. Once you've developed your acuity, your ability to discern and discriminate between the two will be greatly enhanced.

❧ ❧ ❧

❦ CHAPTER TWENTY ❧

The Third Partner

*"Nothing we ever imagined is beyond our power,
only beyond our present self-knowledge."*
— Theodore Rozak

On the Table

You've activated your hands, you've discovered how the energy feels to you, and you've learned how to play with it and keep it present as you move your hands around. Now you're ready to see what happens when you bring the third partner—the patient—into the equation.

How do you include the patient in the flow of energy between you and the universe? What kinds of responses can you expect—from both the patient and yourself?

Before I answer these questions, let me suggest that at this point it might be easier if your "patient" were an acquaintance who's willing to lie down and let you practice on him or her. Create your initial sessions where neither you nor the other person has any investment in the outcome—one way *or* the other. In other words, practice on someone who is neither attached to having a healing nor determined to *prove you wrong*. I might suggest you simply say to someone, "You know, I'm reading this unusual book. . . . May I see your hand for a moment?" If it's all right with them, hold your hands in position around theirs, begin the "feel for it, find it, stretch it" approach, and once you feel it responsively in your own hands, ask them what they're feeling. There's no need for the person to actually require a healing—although there's always benefit for those involved. Keep it light. The last thing you want is a sense of pressure to "do something" or to perform.

Don't lead them by telling them what you think they should be feeling. Simply play. Feel for it, find it, stretch it. Wait for it to arrive, then move with it. And listen with your hands. Listen . . . with a different sense.

If you're in a more relaxed atmosphere, you may want to have your friend lie down on his or her back on a massage table or whatever other arrangement you've decided on. Have the person close their eyes, and remind them to just *notice,* to withdraw their participatory thought process and simply observe when there's something to notice, as well as when there's nothing to notice; to lie there and let go, as if they had a little unexpected rest time.

I wouldn't suggest that they make their minds a blank or try to think of nothing. As a rule, people have trouble with the concept of thinking of nothing. The mind is always going. Suggest that they simply notice whatever it is that brings itself to their attention. This gives them something to do and has a tendency to alleviate the stress often encountered when trying to think of nothing . . . and finding that you don't know how. Direct them to place their attention inside their bodies and to allow it to travel through them. Observing whatever they perceive as out of the ordinary can give them enough to occupy their minds without them getting lost in mental "shoulds" and "shouldn'ts."

Now you're ready to begin.

Allow Space

As discussed earlier, with Reconnective Healing, a big part of the experience for most patients is the various sensations they'll have during the session. But there's a benefit in this for the healer as well, and that's that almost all patients will display visible registers as you work with them. Some patients will also hear, see, or smell things that no one else in the room is aware of. You don't want to interfere with this process in any way, which is, as I've said before, the reason you should avoid wearing loose clothing that may dangle onto the patient with your every movement; letting your hair fall onto the patient, touching the patient's own hair, face, or body inadvertently; wearing or using scents in the room; humming or playing music; or even casting random shadows on the patient's eyelids. With this in mind, it's time to play again—only this time with a companion.

Moving Along the Body

First, position yourself near the patient's body. How close should you stand? After I establish my connection with the patient's field, I find that I like to bring my hands anywhere from one to several feet away from their body. Does the energy change when I pull farther out? Yes. It gets *stronger!* Why should that be? *I don't know!*

Move in and out from your patient, remaining cognizant and in touch with your sensations, as you observe the responses of the person on your table. Although this person has their eyes closed, you as facilitator are to leave your eyes open during Reconnective Healing sessions. Your eyes are an integral part of the healing process, and they have far more of a purpose than to simply notice the perpendicularity of the walls.

Explore while you follow the energy. Let it guide you. Observe how the registers are affected by your movement. Observe how their changes correspond with the differences in intensity and character you feel in and around your hands. As you become more comfortable with it, you'll start to notice registers of feeling—internal registers of dynamic response—occurring within your own body as well.

What part of the patient's body should you work with first. The head? The hands? Should you start by working with a specific chakra? It truly doesn't matter. I often start at the head or chest area. It's also not uncommon to begin at the feet. It varies depending upon instinct, and is often influenced by my angle of approach. In other words, don't give it much more conscious attention than you would when approaching a chair from the left or right side. The more premeditated analysis you give it, the more you distance yourself from finding the "groove."

If you choose to start at the top, stand so that you can comfortably place one hand on each side of the patient's head, arms relaxed and extended in normal anatomic position. Now find the energy—or more appropriately stated, let the energy find you. Again, feel for it, find it, stretch it. Feel the tingle, or heat, or cold, or whatever it is for *you*. Don't concern yourself with whether you're feeling the right thing. Whatever sensation you have is the appropriate one. *It's not* what *you feel; it's that* you feel. Once it's there, work it a bit—stretch the taffy or slink the Slinky.

Now, leaving your hands in a relaxed position, move them in and out easily, or move them around in small circles. Mix, match, and combine until you find the confluence. This is the rhythm of your life. Your energy is now coming into a different realm, and your being will recognize a greater depth of perception, and integrate that force into your existence. You are finding the rhythm that amplifies the wavelength, which amplifies the force coming through you. That gauge, that dial, to amplify that energy, is in your life and in your control.

I often begin by rotating my hands in a vertical plane if I'm by the head or feet, or in a horizontal plane if I'm over the body. Or, I might let one or both hands wander in exploratory movements. Don't overanalyze it; just allow your hands to move and explore according to your instinct.

What you're doing here is developing a contact or communication between your energetic field and that of the patient. You're joining your energy with theirs, and with that of the rest of the universe. Not only can the patient feel it, but you'll often be able to feel in one hand, the movement of your other hand.

For instance, imagine someone lying on their back on a table, you standing on their left facing them. With your left hand facing palm down, move it in a small circular pattern over an area above their legs, allowing for a steady buildup of sensation to come into your hand. Now stretch it up just a little and hold it in its pulled intensity. Take your right hand and locate a spot half a foot or so above the person's chest. Again, start to explore it with a small, circular motion; and stretch it upward. As you maintain the "pull" or "stretch" in each hand, notice that you can strongly detect the circular pattern your right hand is making in an energy swirling in the palm of your left hand. As you reach this elevated degree of sensitivity, you become aware of new levels in the feedback loop. This is the next step of your advancement toward mastery, as feedback is highly instrumental at this point. It is of your being that these energies flow through you. You are not only a part, but a participant, in this exchange. It's not outside you; it's *inside* you.

For the first time, you're involving someone else's energy in the process. What you're feeling is a confluence—and this confluence is allowing you to experience a greater depth of perception, not only during healing sessions, but in your life.

There's No Interference

A key word above is *confluence*. Another illuminating word is *essence*. Older, more solid matter-based perspectives of the world, along with their perception of limitations brought about by our supposed four-dimensional existence, might tell you that a person's physical body will block or impede energy flow. Often you see evidence of "healers" buying into this illusion when they turn the person over or around to "get to the other side." There *is* no other side. This is a *fear-based* illusion. The living human being before you is in no way an interference with the flow of reconnective energy. In actuality, they are an integral part of the interaction. Their essence is the component that brings this new confluence into existence. Not only does the person contribute, but he or she couldn't block the energy if they played major league football.

If this is getting a little "out there" for you, let me explain from a physics perspective. If you extracted all the empty space from a human body, the resulting chunk of matter would be proportionate to a golf ball sitting in an empty football field. Or think about it this way: If you expanded a hydrogen atom to the size of that same football field, the nucleus would be the golf ball, while the electron would be orbiting around at the distance to the end zone. In between is nothing but empty space—plenty of room to allow the energy from one of your hands to make its way to the other one.

Do What Feels Right

At this point, you and the patient are sharing the same energy. Start making your way slowly along their body. Allow your hands to continue moving in and out with the energy. In which direction do you travel? In whichever one feels right to you. How do you move your hands: Do you do circles, do you stretch, do you float them? Let your hands tell you that. You're interacting with life force. Your energy is existing in a sphere of influence that is central to your understanding of a *different* sphere of influence. You are carrying its force in a varied and multidimensional way.

You're a receiver. This is not a conscious, decision-making process. It's like when you walk somewhere. You know you're moving from this point to that one, but you don't think, *Okay, I'm going to lift my left foot and put down the heel, then the toe; now I'm going to shift my weight forward and lift up the right foot and put down the heel, then the toe . . .* you just walk.

If you're having any trouble detaching, let's recall an exercise from a few chapters back. Again imagine that you're talking to someone on the telephone. Now bring your eyes up a little and off to one side. You are listening intently. Remember? *Listen* with your hands. *Just* pay attention—don't think about what you feel. Don't analyze it. Don't interpret it. Just feel.

For illustrative purposes, I'll share what *I* might do during a typical healing session. I might begin at the foot of the table, making a circular motion with one hand toward the soles of the patient's feet. It might feel to me as if I'm stirring something up, although the truth is, I don't know why this is so often where I begin a session. I'm not conscious of making the choice, and with equal frequency, I may begin over the stomach area or at the top of the head. The circular or stirring movement heightens my awareness of the initial sensation, as you might wiggle your toes a little as you first dip them into a lake or pool.

I'll often start by looking for areas over the patient's body that give me the most feedback or sensation. The person's eyes might still be open, and we'll chat as I move one hand in a circular motion, while the other hand is pulling or pushing. Finally, I'll ask the patient to close their eyes and relax, and I'll continue on from there.

Your Right Hand Knows What Your Left Hand Is Doing

By the way, I rarely move both my hands synchronously. When you do that, you're just creating patterns for patterns' sake. How do you know this? Think about windshield wipers—they move either parallel to one another or in opposition, but always in a steady, synchronized manner. This pattern works because windshield wipers can treat all raindrops in the same way. But it's not what's most appropriate for *us*. One area or location might feel one way to us, while another will feel different. Since each has unique characteristics, we are not being true to the process if we disregard this fact and simply move for movement's sake.

Let's say you're sitting in a darkened movie theater. Your drink is on the floor by your left foot, and your popcorn is in a bag in your friend's lap, who's seated on your right. Close your eyes now and feel for your drink and popcorn at the same time. Notice how your right and left hands move in two unrelated fashions. This is because you're actually taking the time to move into the sensation, allowing your hands to respond individually to sensory feedback from two objects of different location, density, and structure. If your hands were both following the same movement patterns, your friend would be wearing the popcorn, and the people seated in front of you would be wearing your soda. You can also think of a pianist or guitar player, whose hands each do something different, yet work together to produce a single, harmonious result.

Similarly, as you move alongside the patient, "listen" with your hands, being alert to variations in the feel of the energy. When you find the energy to be stronger or weaker or in some other way unusual, play with it—stretch it, move it, interact with it. Notice if it feels bubbly, like the jet from a Jacuzzi or the carbonation of club soda; cool and airy like a generalized breeze; or hot and delineated, as if you'd just dropped your fingertips into hot wax. Whatever in the patient's energy attracts your attention, stop and play with it—but not with any specific goals in mind. Focus on the process, not the result. Just play with it as long as it feels interesting and stimulating to you. Then move on.

Meanwhile, pay attention to the rest of the patient's body. Watch the patient's eyes without losing sight of the rest of them. To the best of your ability, be aware of all changes, and correlate these responses with what you're feeling in your hands at the same time.

This is very important, because it ensures that you don't confuse random or imagined sensations in your hands with authentic energy flow and connection.

Common Registers

As I've mentioned previously, a register is an involuntary physical or physiologic response to the frequencies. These registers are as varied and random as the sensations we experience during the healing sessions. There is no one single register to expect. Some patients register more strongly than others—but chances are that something will make itself evident in the patient as you establish your connection. As you move your hands, exploring and discovering more of the intricacies of this communication, the registers will vary not only in intensity, but in character. At seminars, some people illustrate this strongly enough so that people in the back of an auditorium can clearly see it, while other volunteers display it so mildly that I can only point it out to the nearest few rows of attendees. Once you and your patient entrain with the energies, chances are that you will start to see these registers clearly.

Whatever the register or response, allow yourself to be okay with *not* defining or assigning meaning to it. These are automatic responses, many as reflexive as the jerk of a knee under a doctor's rubber mallet. Tears could indicate joy as much as sorrow, or the release of pain. A register is best thought of as an indication that you've found a good "spot" in the energy field—a connected place to be.

You'll notice that the more you work with an area that has brought about a register, the more the patient tends to exhibit that register. And when the register slows down, or your interest in that specific register begins to wane, move on and find another. What do these involuntary displays mean? Registers are an indication that the person on the table has gone to the place where decisions are made regarding their healing.

There are three things which, on the surface, appear to have nothing to do with one another: the location of the person's symptoms, the place where you hold your hands, and the area of the person's registers. In other words, registers will frequently not correspond at all with the area of the body where the patient's injury or ailment is thought to exist.

For example, working near the feet might result in a person's headache leaving them, as much as working near the head might bring about the same response. Working near the head might result in a person's hearing being restored as easily as it might result in their bunions vanishing. Also, their registers could manifest in their knees as readily as on their face. It doesn't matter where you stand or where you hold your hands. Your function is to find an interesting place in the patient's energy field, and play with it until you feel like moving on. Why an interesting place? Because when your interest is heightened, it keeps you present and connected. And each time you go to a new place on the body, you re-present and re-connect.

Yes, that's really all you do. Feel the energy in a spot, then *play with it, discover it, explore it*—without expectations or goals. The energy has its resonance in your hands and in your inner life. It is circular in nature. Bring your hands closer together or farther away, rotate them in circles, and do whatever feels right or enhances your connection at the time. Don't flail about or make "pretty" patterns in the air just for the sake of moving. Keep full awareness of the sensations you're perceiving in relation to the registers in the patient. You'll notice that the more you work with the spot, the more the register is exhibited . . . or the more other registers tend to join the symphony. You are orchestrating this energy in a manner that is befitting of a kind of "harmonic convergence" within the lives you're touching.

Following are a few of the more common registers.

Rapid Eye Movement (REM)

Rapid eye movement, which is often the initial register for a person, represents a fascinating dichotomy because, although the patient often experiences that incredible state of stillness, from the outside, he or she appears to be anything *but* still. It's similar in appearance to what happens when a sleeping person moves into the dream state. But in the case of a person having a reconnective experience, the cause is clearly different because, once again, the patient is *not* asleep. The REM that occurs with the reconnective frequencies tends to take on a number of distinct patterns. Sometimes it's a light eyelid flutter, but other times it's a strong one. Sometimes it's rapid, sometimes slow. Usually it's steady, but sometimes the pattern is difficult to discern. In half the people, it's the eyelids that are moving; in the other half, it's the eye itself. Sometimes when the eye is moving, it's a slow, almost wandering motion; other times it's a rapid darting, back and forth. Sometimes, one or both eyes partially open; usually, they both remain closed. Almost always, the eyes show a register. Whether REM or not, the patient is most often fully aware of what's going on.

Breathing Changes

Breathing changes are one of the initial registers, generally occurring just after or simultaneously with the eye register. There are many ways in which this register might manifest itself: faster, deeper, or irregular breathing; and what I call "puff breathing." I came up with this term to refer to a type of unusual respiration that occurs when the lips are relaxed and slightly parted, so that each breath escapes with a soft, gentle *poof* of air. Side-mouth breathing is a variation on puff-breathing, where the "puffing" occurs at the corner of one's mouth. There's also snoring—which differs from the traditional form only in that the patient is awake, and aware of making the sound.

Sometimes a person will stop breathing altogether! Believe it or not, this is a desirable response, a heightened state of unity in which you can experience the stillness and the silence of the universe. The breathing will resume at the appropriate moment.

There's a thread of continuity running through all of these breathing changes. The Vedic term *samadhi* refers to a oneness, a state of unity and bliss. It is in this state that one often reports being neither awake nor asleep,

yet being somewhere more real than either one. This is what is reported
by many who experience these alterations in consciousness, these alterations
in breathing. Although they may not know the term *samadhi,* these patients
describe a very similar state, and they're often aware through parts of it of
the changes and unusual patterns in their breathing.

You walk a fine line in certain situations. You don't want to color someone's experience by telling them what they might expect; on the other hand,
you don't want unexpected experiences to jolt them out of their sessions.
Most people are in such a blissful state by the time they experience these
breathing changes that they simply enjoy the ecstasy of it. Once in a while,
someone's logical mind will get in their way, though. They'll realize they've
stopped breathing, and although the experience is beautifully exquisite, they
try to force themselves to breathe again. If this is what they report to you
after a session, let them know for future reference that they are perfectly
safe in that place and they need not attempt to force themselves to resume
breathing. In the course of a healing, sometimes your breathing stops for
a while because your experience is *supposed* to include a moment of complete stillness, a reflection of your total connection to the "oneness" you're
experiencing. When it's time for your patient to breathe again, they will.
They just will.

Swallowing

Swallowing tends to be third in the initial grouping of registers. Often
there is an increase in the frequency and/or intensity of the person's swallowing. Sometimes it lasts throughout most of the session; usually it's only
present during the earlier portion. It's a very common register and usually
kicks in, if it's going to, within the first few minutes of the session, yet
shows up somewhat less often and with less intensity than the REM and
breathing registers.

Tears

Also, the sudden appearance of tears is a fascinating register. Seemingly without warning, the tears will well up in a person's eyes, spill over,
and stream ceaselessly down their cheeks while the patient's facial expres-

sion remains one of bliss. The tears are a reaction to touching Truth, to experiencing and remembering Truth. It's recognizing Truth as the place where we all come from and the place to which we'll all return, the place we haven't seen for what seems like a very long time. When we receive the honor of touching Truth and interacting with it, even for a moment, it brings up our emotions because of that sense of being Home, and knowing we'll be there again soon.

Laughter

Sometimes the person on your table will break into uncontrollable laughter. They'll most likely tell you that they don't know why they're laughing. It's good to let them know that it's okay to laugh. If they don't feel that it's acceptable, it will make them laugh all the more, and it may interfere with the experiential aspect of their session. Verbally giving them permission to laugh, once it starts, will generally diffuse it.

Finger Movements

A register which, for many, waits several minutes into the session before starting, is finger movement. Involuntary finger movements tend to occur bilaterally, synchronously, or asynchronously. Sometimes the fingers of both hands will move, sometimes just one. Sometimes the fingers of both hands may move simultaneously; other times the fingers of one hand will move, then the other hand will follow. As the session progresses, you'll often see the hand and wrist become involved. For some people, the arm will also involve itself. Variations on this pattern occur with the feet as well.

Head Rotation and Body Movements

Sometimes the head will slowly roll or feel pulled to one side and/or the other.

Commonly seen body movements relate to the abdomen and the chest. You will also see the arms and/or legs "jump."

Stomach Gurgling

Often, people's stomachs "gurgle" or make noise during the sessions, especially when your hands are over that area of the body. I suggest that you let people know, prior to beginning your session, that this is a common occurrence. Some people may be self-conscious about this and, if not told that it is to be expected, may allow it to keep them from enjoying the experience.

Letting Things Take Their Own Course . . . and Your Responsibility

Let me take a moment to discuss letting things take their own course. Although it's true that, from the outside, you can't really interpret accurately what the person on the table is experiencing, this force has its own intelligence—a very High Intelligence. It knows what's appropriate for the person on the table even though our limited, educated, inductively oriented minds may not.

The reconnective sessions are almost always perceived as pleasurable, valuable, and unique. Once in a rare moment, someone may interpret his or her session as otherwise. *Their interpretation of their session is not your responsibility.* You do, however, want to employ a modicum of common sense. As discussed earlier, someone crying on a table or appearing to be in physical distress is generally not experiencing internally what they appear to be externally. People clutching at their hearts, pointing toward the heavens, gasping, "I'm coming, Ethel!" may be deserving of your checking in with them. You will learn to use your own discretion and judgment as to whether or not to interrupt the session.

So far, of the few times I took it upon myself to intervene since all this began in 1993, I was told by my patients that everything was wonderful and that they wanted to continue their sessions.

There may never really be a reason for us to intervene, as this is being mediated by a force beyond our comprehension. Yet, should you choose to do so, a soft word from you will usually open communication, allowing you to check in with the person. If your patient does not respond, you may choose to gently bring them out of their session by lightly—or firmly, if the situation warrants—touching them just below their collarbone (or on their shoulder) and calling them by name. On the rarest of occasions, I've felt the need to simultaneously snap my fingers a couple of times by one of their ears while doing the above. You may want to instruct your patient to open their eyes and keep them open for a few moments until they feel clear. A glass of water placed in close proximity is also helpful.

Once in a while, someone may not recognize a healing. You are not responsible for that, either. It may have come in a form that will make itself apparent later, or it may have come in a form that will not be readily discernible at *any* point in the near future. And, as I mentioned earlier, when asked, "Does everyone have a healing?" I used to say, "No." I no longer feel that way. I feel that everyone *does* have a healing; it's just that it may not arrive with trumpets and bugles.

What You Might Feel

Up to this point in the book, I've referenced only a few of the sensations you might experience in your hands or body. This was to give you some time to make your own discoveries as we moved along. Now I'd like to give you a slightly more expansive list so you may see in print some of what you've no doubt already encountered in your evolution into the transsensory. The relationship and interaction between you and the energies is unique, individual, and very intimate. It's integral that you heighten your awareness and your familiarity with the intricacies of these sensations, because it is from this point of recognition that you begin to develop your artistry. The levels of proficiency this will take you to are indescribable.

Here are some of the more frequently reported practitioner sensations:

Bubbles: A sensation of tiny, little soda bubbles; or marble-sized bubbles; or bubbles the size of a cue or tennis ball may come up into your palm.

Water: This often comes as a sensation of droplets or light rain.

Sparkles: Have you ever wondered what the sparks showering off a Fourth-of-July sparkler would feel like? Well, this is it.

Here are some other common sensations you might experience:

- Dryness
- Heat

- Cold

- Hot, cold, wet, and dry simultaneously
  (I can't explain this one, but once you've felt it,
  you'll know what I mean)

- Pulling

- Pushing

- Throbbing

- Electricity

- Magnetic attraction

- Magnetic repelling

- Air-density changes

- Breezes (usually cool and site-specific)

- Expansion—a feeling of your body being expanded in size—often
  compared to a "space suit" or "air suit" shaped like your body, yet
  frequently much larger. This is sometimes focal in the area of an
  arm or a leg; sometimes specific to one-quarter or one-half of the
  body; other times more comprehensive.

Keep Moving

Continue moving along the patient's body, finding spots in the energy
that you feel like playing with. If you don't feel anything at all, you're probably trying too hard. Just let go and wait. You don't need to go into "performance mode," reaching your hands up over your head and melodra-
matically calling for Spirit or God; you don't need to go into a big production
to bring the feeling back. Just let go and say to yourself, *All right, I'm a
little too focused on this. I'm going to step back and allow the feeling to
come into my hands.* Then let it go. Place your attention back on your hands,
and wait until the sensation returns. It's that simple.

Feel for it, find it, *investigate it!* As your proficiency grows, you can
move fairly quickly. When you find a place, slow down and get to know
it. Maintain the contact. Bring it out, amplify it, work with it. It's sometimes the most intricate explorations that bring about the most powerful

results. You might use both hands over the area, or one hand might wander off to find a second spot—a spot of new interest so that they each have an area to work with. During this process, allow your hands to have a life of their own—their own inquisitiveness.

But remember, you are *not* looking for *preexisting* spots. This is a very important point, a distinction between this new level of healing and evolution, and the limitations and misconceptions of some of the earlier "technique" approaches.

In the past, you might have attended classes where the healer/instructor said they were going to teach you "scanning." Standing over the patient, the instructor would float their hands in the air and say, "Let's see, it's . . . oh, here it is, it's right here. Now, everyone get in line and see if you can feel it. Can you feel it there? Good. Next. Can you feel it there? Good. Next . . ."

Well, that's *not* "it," and it's *not* "there." There is no fixed "spot" to feel. Remember, a healing does not consist of a patient there on the table and a healer hovering over him or her, directing energy into their body or looking for a preexisting area of congestion. These transformations are an equation—and as with any equation, if you change the numbers, you're going to get different answers. Similarly, if two people try to find the same spot, they won't both find it—*because the spot isn't there.*

Discovery, as science points out, may well be an act of *creation*. The spot that appears for *me* is not the spot that makes itself known to *you*. The spot is a joint creation, a product of love and feeling and communication between you, the patient, and the universe. There emerges from this triad a conveyance: the eternal and formless essence of our ever-evolving universe.

Omnidirectional Connection Points

Having said that, let me add that particular areas of the body tend to elicit the strongest registers. You are still creating the *spots*, yet you may be going to more fertile areas in the field. You're likely to get the greatest responses while playing with the energy in the vicinity of the top of the head (what's commonly called the *crown chakra*); the center of the forehead (what's known as the *third eye* area); the throat; the heart; the lower abdomen; the backs or tops of the hands and wrists; and the tops of the feet and the soft spots over the ankles. I call these highly responsive areas *connection points*. Accessing, connecting, and communicating with a person's field can be very easy from these points, and often reveal more highly demonstrable registers. You can think of them as "hubs" where information is exchanged.

A Multi-tiered, Reciprocal, Dynamic Feedback System

The feedback you'll receive from the patient on the table goes beyond the registers mentioned above. It's not only multi-tiered, it's dynamic and reciprocal. On one tier, there you are. You're stretching the energy, for example. You feel the sensation. Then, as you pull it up, the patient's eyes move a certain way. That's the register. But at the same time, you feel an intensity shift in *your* sensations. That's how you know that what you were doing was *responsible* for the eye shift.

On one level of feedback, the patient has an external response. On another level, there might not be a visible response, yet you have an internal reaction in your hands or body. Yet, when you combine the two, there's a *dynamic* feedback system that allows for more fine-tuning. It's more than feeling something and noticing the person's response. It's you being "in tune," allowing yourself to feel what's going on, and noticing at the moment of a shift (a clear, recognizable shift) in your feeling or sensation, that *boom!*—there's a simultaneous change or specific response in the patient.

You're moving into an alert state of awareness. Further refinements will let you, when using your hands independently, feel in one hand what the *other* hand is doing! In other words, you might come in on a "track" with your left hand and find a certain spot, then track in with your right hand and find a second spot. You circle your right hand there, then become aware of that circular motion in your left hand, which is not circling. When you do this, it seems to further intensify the field around the person, and you start to develop stronger registers in the patient.

You can tell not only from what you're doing, but from what you're seeing and feeling in *relation* to what you're doing, that the new level of intensity you found for yourself correlates to a heightened and more dramatic response in the patient. Often, you seem to get stronger reactions with smaller movements. Just when you feel lost in the ecstasy, suddenly the patient's arm or knee will take a "leap." It's like a subatomic particle *here,* responding simultaneously to the movement of a subatomic particle *there.* This is one of the premises upon which distance healing, absentee healing, and remote healing function.

As you continue to watch the patient, perhaps you don't see much move-ment or notice any change of sensation in your own hands. You continue to look around, and *boom* again!—there's a big eye-flip or other register, and at the same moment, the *patient* feels something in *their* hands.

You must accept the fact that some patients show far more registers than others. That doesn't mean that the healing is better or worse than some other healing. Nor does it mean that it's more or less effective. It's like buy-ing two cars. One's got every imaginable gauge on the panel—RPM, oil pressure, engine temp, brake fluid level—you name it. The second car is an older vehicle, and its instrument panel tells you when the radiator is over-heating or when you're low on gas, and that's it.

Here's the point: Just because you're getting less feedback from the old car, that doesn't mean it's not running as well as the new one. So don't assess what you're doing based on what you see.

Still, you need to develop sensitivity, a type of artistry of touch, in order to recognize the "feel." Keep your vision on the patient's main kick-in reg-ister sites, such as their eyes, their breathing, or their swallowing; but leave your vision peripheral, too, to catch signs—indicators that might appear in their fingers, toes, or anywhere else. At the same time, learn to recog-nize the sensations that go with the movements. This is your multi-tiered, reciprocal, dynamic feedback system.

Let's pretend you're driving an automatic car. With your foot, you *feel for* and *find* the gas pedal. You're now setting up the beginning of a feed-back system. When you push on the gas pedal and the car begins to accel-erate, you're now merging into the feedback system. The sensory recep-tors in your foot create a feedback system that continually tells you how much dynamic pressure and tension you're maintaining on the accelera-tor. The acceleration of the car gives you different feedback about the amount of pressure and tension you're maintaining on the accelerator.

Because you have two sets of feedback, the system is *multi-tiered*. Because each affects the other, the system is *reciprocal*. And because receiv-ing feedback is a continuing process that changes with variation in either acceleration or pressure on the accelerator, the system is *dynamic*. You are now in a *multi-tiered, reciprocal, dynamic feedback system*. At a certain point, you pick up speed, the automatic transmission will "shift" into another gear, and you will feel the subtle lurching-forward of the vehicle.

You have, at that point, entered into a relationship with another feed-back system, while remaining in the original multi-tiered reciprocal dynamic system. Not only are you receiving feedback about your pressure and tension on the accelerator from both the sensory system of your foot and from the acceleration of the car, you're also receiving it from the pressure of your body against your seat back. You now have three tiers of feedback giving you information about the pressure and tension on the accelerator. Even your visual feedback, which has been operating simultaneously with all of this, has to take in multiple tiers as you evaluate speed by both stationary objects, such as trees; and nonstationary objects, such as birds and other vehicles—all of which are moving at different speeds.

When your automatic transmission "shifts" into another gear, you register a body jerk as the car makes a not-so-subtle and more perceptible lurch forward. You register a pressure change with the accelerator, and your brain must, once again, take into account, and compensate for, visual reference point changes (vehicles, birds, trees, and so on.). You are in a feedback system within a feedback system within feedback systems.

Let's pretend you've bought a new car, with manual transmission—and you only know how to drive an automatic. Now you not only have to account for the entirety of the above feedback system, you have to incorporate knowing *how*, and knowing *when,* to shift, developing a new learning curve that initially takes into account shifting according to RPM gauges, later to be superseded by shifting by sound and other newly developed and refined internal gauges. This is but one of many multi-tiered reciprocal dynamic feedback systems we work with every day. It is a *learned* system, just as is the one in this book. You're developing a *learning curve* because, although much of the feedback is subtle, it's *real—like the University of Arizona study.*

Just as we learn to discriminate depth as an infant and learn to perceive the difference between a window, a painting, a mirror, and an opening in a wall leading into another room, we can learn to perceive these energies. All of these things are real. None are fabricated—although, to the uninitiated, they may appear so. And none of these energies, once recognized and automatic, or "second nature" (a term I now find fascinating)—*are* subtle. Just like my point.

❧ ❧ ❧

❧ CHAPTER ❧
TWENTY-ONE
Interacting with Your Patients

*"The most powerful thing you can do to change the world is
to change your own beliefs about the nature of life, people, reality,
to something more positive . . . and begin to act accordingly."*
— from *Creative Visualization,* by Shakti Gawain

You Are Your Instrument

You've now developed your ability to recognize when reconnective energy is flowing through you. You know how to spot registers, you're familiar with the "feel" of the energy around a patient's body, and you're now comfortable playing with this energy and letting what's going to happen, happen.

In other words, you're ready to be of assistance to someone in their healing.

Remember, your main goal in a Reconnective Healing session is to get yourself out of the way. As your body continues in its shift and accommodation to carry the new frequencies, and after you've developed some familiarity with the feedback that's part of using these energies, you'll find that everything falls into place. Still, you'll want to cultivate a certain mind-set before you begin working with other human beings. After all, now that you've hopefully kicked your old "healing toy" dependency, the only "instrument" you'll be using for this kind of healing is *you.*

🖋 🖋 🖋

Words to Heal By

Remain in awe.

How can you remain in awe? By being childlike. By seeing everything through new eyes. By not being so quick to presume to understand what you're witnessing. The understanding you presume is most likely some surface explanation passed on to you via countless filtrations and misinterpretations, leaving it thin, watery, and without substance. Know that your one connection to this mind-set, which no one can sever, is your ability to say, "I don't know." With this, you have the faculty to view everything with genuine wonder.

Do you remember the gift of being childlike and being in awe of everything?

Remember this gift!

The gift of being in awe, of viewing everything with genuine wonder, gives your reverence the crystalline purity of childhood, an inherent connection to God. It releases your desire to diagnose, to explain, to try, to make, to force, to push, to exert effort. It even releases your need to take credit.

Now do you remember this gift?

This is the time to get your heart, mind, and intentions in order. You're about to become part of a healing equation.

"Prepping" the Patient

As a rule, new patients fall into one of two groups. There are those who arrive at your office, lie down on the table, and let go, hoping to experience whatever comes their way. Then there are those who hit the table running, doing everything possible that they think they "should" be doing during their session. Their minds are going a mile a minute. They're praying, visualizing, repeating mantras, breathing from their stomach, breathing from their chest, keeping their palms up, meditating, holding their hands in a prayer position, and so on.

Their lips are moving faintly, with tears streaming—sometimes silently, sometimes in conjunction with wails, while inside they're asking God for everything they might want for themselves and possibly everyone else they know. Left unchecked, this monologue and assortment of processes will go on for the length of the entire visit, and this person will have cheated themselves out of the experiential aspect of the reconnective session. It will be the same as if they had been in a prayer group, a technique-type healing session, or simply meditating at home.

You're not going to want this to happen. But you're also not going to want to tell them what *not* to do prior to their doing it. That's like saying, "Don't picture the color red." So what you want to do when you see you've got a potential *doer* or *chatterer* on the table is head them off at the pass.

Here's what I might say to them: "Come in. Lie down, close your eyes. Let yourself drift, without falling asleep. Trust that whoever it is that hears your thoughts and prayers has already heard yours. Not only have they heard what you've already asked for, they've also heard what you *haven't* thought to ask for. They've known all along. Even before you walked in. So stop talking, stop the mind chatter, and just listen; let the universe bring you whatever it decides you need. Just lie there and be as open to experiencing *nothing* as you are to experiencing *something*. In that openness, your experience will arrive."

This is not easy advice for many people to follow, but it's the best advice you can give them. Optimally, they'll just let go and lie there without expectation. It's desirable for them to be in a state of expectancy, open to receiving *something*. The balancing act is to not cross over into a state of expectation, where their focus shifts onto what the exact result should be. One, because that might not be what they really need, or what the universe has in mind for them in their best interests; and two, fixed expectations may constrict, limit, or replace what might otherwise come their way.

Similarly, it's up to you to be receptive and nonjudgmental, also—to wait and be part of what's going to happen—whatever it might be. Waiting is a form of "listening with spirit." You wait until the energy arrives. Which it does. And all of a sudden, it's running through the patient and connected *with* you, *through* you, and *around* you.

It's not for us to determine what type of healing a person needs to experience. It's our task to offer ourselves as part of the equation and to let the healing take its own natural form.

As part of the nonjudgmental approach I described earlier, I usually don't become attached to the specific problem a patient comes in with. I let them talk about it to a point because it helps them feel bonded with me, which can be important. But the truth is, whether you know what's wrong with a patient or not, they're going to experience the same healing. I believe there's an intelligence in the universe that's involved in this, an intelligence far beyond yours or mine, and the appropriate healing will manifest itself.

Let It Be

The need for us to keep our egos out of the equation goes deeper than you might expect. For example, many healing practitioners want to focus their minds on the *how*—something as seemingly innocuous as picturing the patient "being healthy," or bringing energy up through their feet, down through their heads, or out through their noses; placing the patient in violet light, or enveloping them in pink clouds . . . trying to project health onto the patient in any way they think might assist. Why? Because this is what they have heard or been told to do in the past. Doubt has already entered here. All of these things are just different forms of interference. The more you try to *do*, the less you're able to *be*—and it's that state of being that allows the energy to flow through you in the first place. The state of being is what gets our *self* out of the way, enabling our *Self* to become part of the process. It's while we're in this state that the healing arrives.

We've been raised to take control of and direct our own lives. Once we've determined the ways in which we feel things "should" be done, the idea of suddenly changing our methods can be frightening. Here's an example.

My great-grandmother, Annie Smith, owned a luncheonette in a predominantly Catholic neighborhood. At that time, Catholics were not permitted to eat meat on Fridays, so every Friday, she made what became her famous fishcakes: mashed potatoes, onions, salt, pepper, special seasonings, and cod—dipped in breadcrumbs and deep-fried to perfection.

There was always a line of people outside her luncheonette waiting for these fishcakes, but on this particular Friday evening, the line extended around the block. All day long, the more people she served, the longer the line seemed to get.

"Hey, Annie, these are the best fishcakes you've ever made," came the raves. Her supply dwindling, Annie sold out and closed the restaurant for the night. My great-grandmother, who stood four and one-half feet tall and was a hard-working dynamo, went into the kitchen to do a final cleaning. While she was putting things away, she opened the refrigerator and was shocked to see that the large bowl of cleaned and boned fish she had so carefully prepared for the cakes was still in there. My great-grandmother had forgotten to add in the fish. She was horrified. She had been serving these people nothing but fried mashed potatoes, onions, and seasoning. How was it that they received such praise: fishcakes that had no fish in them? The closest anyone got to fish that day was the aroma coming off the counter and some possible residue from the mixing pots. What she had sold, in part, was the *essence* of fishcakes. Annie never told anyone, and the following Friday, she went back to adding the cod. Might Annie's fishless fishcakes, which she could have sold along with her regular fishcakes, have become the new toast of the town? We'll never know. This story is an example of how someone might be shown something different, or be given a choice to step out of their comfort zone, yet quite often, they will remain in—or in this case—go back to, what was the known.

Sometimes we're shown new ways. Sometimes we have the courage to follow them.

Bedside Manner

Another aspect of keeping your ego out of the equation is to maintain a healthy state of detachment—not becoming too involved in your patient's process. As discussed earlier, the person on the table is most likely in a state of stillness and bliss, often with involuntary body movements. On rare occasions, as mentioned previously, tears may suddenly appear. This is not an invitation for you to step in with a hug and soothing words. Please resist our culturally reinforced impulse to interfere in that fashion. This is the *patient's* experience, and it is part of their process. Do not deprive them of this. More than likely, and despite outward appearances, they are enjoying what's going on. If you feel compelled to do something, gently ask them if they're okay or if they'd like to end the session. Odds are that they'll tell you that they're just fine. If they want to bring themselves out of it, they most likely will. As I've said before, if someone wants your assistance in coming out of a session, a light touch, calling their name, and a nearby glass of water should do the trick.

Stay sensitive and available should this unexpected situation arise. It will be up to you to assist the patient—not just as a healer, but as a caring human being. In these cases, simply reassure the patient that everything's fine, that such reactions are normal and acceptable, and in their case, probably even necessary. When they've calmed down, you can continue, or postpone the treatment to another time—whichever feels right to all involved.

〰 〰 〰

Falling Asleep

You want your patients to "check out" and not think or worry about what's happening as they lie on the table, but sometimes the checking out goes too far and the patient falls asleep. This is not my favorite way to work. I innately get the feeling that a sleeping patient may not be getting the full benefit of the healing process. Not to mention that the part of me that is ego wants the patient to have enjoyed the conscious experiential aspect.

However, realize that if the patient sleeps during the session, it's what's appropriate for that person. Also, if a patient is just too active for you to handle in any other way—that is, someone who is hyperactive (or a child), by all means do the work while they're asleep.

What about you, the healer? Is it possible for *you* to fall asleep during a session? Yes, but usually that's indicative of the fact that you haven't been getting enough sleep, and/or you're not "in the moment." Either way, please honor the patient and the situation by taking care of your own needs so you can be there for them. I am reminded of the safety precaution one is given on airplanes: *Mothers, please place the oxygen mask on yourself before placing it on your child.*

Remember, you're allowing your mind to reach a place where you're not exactly awake and not exactly asleep—where you're somewhere else. This is the place where healing energy comes to Earth.

Debriefing the Patient

> *A wise old bird sat in an oak.*
> *The more he heard, the less he spoke.*
> *The less he spoke, the more he heard.*
> *Why don't you be like that wise old bird?*
> — Author unknown

For those of you who intend to keep records—and I encourage you to do so, if not for yourselves, then at least so you can send me material for my upcoming books!—there is an art to what I call "debriefing" the patient. Believe it or not, the patient looks at you as an authority figure and wants to please you. If you let them know, consciously or unconsciously, what type of answers you want, those are the answers you're going to get. In order to get accurate information, keep good records, and hopefully not skew your data, my suggestion is as follows.

At the end of the session, gently touch the person just below their collarbone and softly let them know that the session is over. When they open their eyes, have your pen and paper or file card (with their name, address, phone numbers, and other information already on it) ready to take notes. It is up to you to direct this part of the session, and I strongly suggest you do so. You might proceed as follows.

1. Ask the patient: *What was your experience?* or *What do you recall?* As they answer your questions, make sure they keep to the facts: *I felt this, I saw that, I heard this, I smelled that.*

2. Have the patient describe in detail what they remember. If they saw a man in a white coat, ask them to describe him. Invite them to remember on their own, phrasing your questions in a nondirective fashion such as: *What else do you recall about him?* Let the patient talk, then ask them questions about hair color, height, length of coat, and what age he appeared. As they continue, help them express or recall as much as they can about each experience.

    Be careful not to lead. An example of leading would be asking if the man was tall, if he had dark hair, or if he appeared to be in his 30s. If the person is somewhat hazy, this type of prompting may unduly affect their memory. After you feel you've gotten all the information you can on the man, ask: *What else do you recall?* "What else" is a good way to phrase it because it invites the patient to look inside their own consciousness for other details. Asking: *"Do you recall anything else?"* is not the same question. You've put it into a yes/no context, and when you phrase things in this manner, the natural tendency, especially in the restful state they're most likely in following a session, is to answer with a *"No."*

3. After you've gotten all the answers—and related details to your "What else?" questions, pose additional queries relating to the five senses: *Was there anything else you saw? Heard? Felt? Smelled? Tasted?* (Yes, on occasion some people even have a "taste" aspect to their sessions.) I like to ask people if I touched them anywhere during the session. If they answer,

for example, "You touched me on my foot," I ask them to show me how I did it. Why? Because "touch" can mean different things to different people. For some people, it means a quick, one-fingered touch; to others, it means a "squeeze" or lightly stroking with two fingers. Once you see what "touch" means, you can more accurately describe it in your notes.

Some Notes for You

Here are a couple of "notes" for *you*. First, at the end of the visit, keep the patient focused on what they *actually experienced during their session*. At this point, don't let them give you their interpretation of what their experience means to them, how it relates to what's going on in their lives, or tell you about their previous experiences they've had somewhere else. If they begin to do so, bring them back to the specifics of *this* experience without interpretation. Why? First of all, their interpretation of what a man in a white coat means is usually little more than a retelling of someone else's idea of what it means, something someone told them or that they read in a book. It's often their way of impressing you with what they think they know, and most likely has little to do with accurate insight into the reality of what they just experienced.

More important, every second the patient spends giving you their impressions, they're forgetting details of what actually occurred for them in this session. For this same reason, you don't want to be sharing any of *your* stories with them at this time. Politely suggest that they remain focused on reporting what actually took place, and let them know that they can give you their interpretations and other stories at the end of this debriefing. If you're lucky, they'll forget.

Here's something else: You may not know how important certain notes may prove to be until quite some time after you've written them. If I didn't take notes the first time one of my patients saw "Parsillia" or "George" or some of the others, I wouldn't have had them to compare to when these beings made themselves known at later dates to other patients.

Also, maintain a poker face. I don't mean a stone face. Be comforting and genuinely interested; just don't show excitement in response to certain types of patient responses over others. If you "light up" every time your patient says they saw someone, in their subconscious attempt to please you, they may find themselves unintentionally embellishing the story with things they "might" be remembering. Then, if you don't exhibit the same degree of "interest" in the next thing that's recalled, they may have a tendency to skip over some of the important details. This is an unconscious way of skewing your own data.

Wait until the end of the session to begin debriefing. Asking them to report things as they occur, unless you have a specific reason, isn't fair to the patient. It interrupts the continuity and depth of the session, depriving them of the fullness of the experiential aspect. The two suggestions I do make prior to starting the session are that, if something they sense in the room gets their attention, they may gently open their eyes to quiet their curiosity, then close them again so that they may continue with their session.

I don't suggest what that something might be because, if they *do* have an experience, I don't want to have unintentionally influenced it. I also tell them that if something happens during the session that they feel is very important to remember, that they should quietly tell me when it occurs. By doing so, I explain, I can write it down to remind them afterward, and they don't have to consciously try to remember it.

❧ ❧ ❧

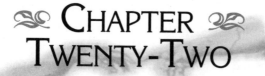

❧ CHAPTER ❧ TWENTY-TWO

What Is Healing?

*"Truth does not change, although your
perception of it may vary or alter drastically."*
— from *Eyes of the Beholder*,
by John and Lyn St. Clair Thomas

If Nothing Seems to Be Happening . . .

If nothing seems to be happening during a session, it's either because you're trying too hard or the patient is. Watch them, and watch their face. If you see motors turning in their head or see them fidgeting, odds are they're doing something on the table other than just "checking out." Usually when I ask what they're doing, they'll say, "Praying." In their mind, they're saying, "Dear Jesus, give me this healing; dear Jesus, give me that healing, God give me this, don't forget that, and I want it to come in this form . . . ," and on and on and on.

I'm not trying to dissuade you or your patient from praying; I'm saying, "Have the faith to be able to say one prayer—*once*—and know that it's been heard.

Self-Healing

People often ask if it's possible to use these energies for healing yourself. Of course it is.

Self-healing is very simple. Almost too simple. Just like distance healing, if you try to make it more complex, it will be less effective.

By now, you're somewhat familiar with the sensation of having the energy moving somewhere in your body. So, find a comfortable place—perhaps a bed or a reclining chair. Be aware that your intention is to enter into the energy for the purpose of self-healing, and acknowledge that fact.

Now allow the sensation of the energy to appear in your hands. Notice as it becomes stronger. Don't try to *force* it; simply *notice* it. *Allow* for it, and wait for it to arrive. It appears when you place your attention on it. As you leave your attention on it, it grows in intensity. The stronger it becomes, the more you notice it. The more you notice it, the stronger it becomes. It's a cycle.

Be aware that as the sensation gets stronger, it also starts to spread. Notice other areas of your body, such as your arms, and wait for the sensation to arrive there—which it will. Then bring your attention into your feet, and notice it start there. Soon it will move up into your legs. As the energy overtakes your body, you begin to vibrate at a higher level. The energy will then become so strong that it starts to block out other sounds and distracting thoughts. Basically, it begins to take over.

Feel it as it takes over, getting larger and larger. Then allow yourself to slip into the gap. No, not the clothing store, the "gap" between your thoughts. As you enter this gap, you are no longer in conscious thought mode. If you're lying there thinking, *I'm healing, I'm healing, I'm healing*—well, "you're not, you're not, you're not." Release the thought.

All of a sudden, you no longer notice anything—because you're *in* the gap. Although you won't notice that either until you've come out of it. Suddenly you open your eyes—five minutes, twenty minutes, an hour and a half later. Or, if you engage in this process late at night, you might choose not to come out of it until the next morning. When it's time for you to come out of the gap, all of a sudden you'll realize you're out. That's it. It's that simple.

Then let it go. Don't come back to it. Know that the appropriate healing has taken place and *walk away*. Why? Because each time you go back for more, you're reinforcing the belief that you *didn't get it all* the first time. *Walk away from it, and don't look back*. This acknowledges in your essence that the healing is full and complete, thus allowing for its totality. Your intention was the prayer. The energy was the communication carrier. Releasing it and not looking back was your thanks and acceptance.

Distance Healing

Richard Gerber, M.D., in his book *Vibrational Medicine*, discusses the Tiller-Einstein Model of positive and negative spacetime: physical matter existing in positive spacetime; energies beyond the speed of light (such as etheric and astral frequencies) existing in negative spacetime. Gerber explains that positive spacetime energy (and matter) are primarily electrical in nature, while negative spacetime energy is primarily magnetic. Accordingly, positive spacetime is also the realm of electromagnetic radiation (EM), while negative spacetime is the realm of magnetoelectric radiation (ME). Negative spacetime energy, aside from its primarily magnetic nature, has another fascinating characteristic: a tendency toward negative entropy. Entropy is a tendency toward disorder, disorganization—*dis*-ease. The higher the entropy, the higher the disorder. Negative entropy is the tendency toward order, organization—ease. It is the tendency toward regeneration and healing.

What does this have to do with distance healing? Reconnective Healing frequencies are not constrained by the laws of positive spacetime. On at least some levels, they are congruent with the concepts of negative spacetime. This is an entirely different reference system. This is probably a partial insight into why there is no reason to use your hands with self-healing or distance healing, and why there is no actual need to use your hands when you are physically present in the room with your patient.

As already discussed, one of the tenets of quantum mechanics is that forces actually become stronger with distance. Working with someone who's not physically present with you gives you the opportunity to experience this phenomenon.

✿ ✿ ✿

To begin the process of distance healing, find a comfortable spot. Close your eyes if you'd like and, as discussed previously in the "Self-Healing" section, allow the sensations to come over you: from your hands into your arms; from your feet into your legs; into your body, and into your being. Consciously become your essence, and be with the person you're connecting with—either in what you envision as their physical environment, or somewhere out into space or blackness, the void—everything and nothing. Know that you're there, and that the other person is there with you. It doesn't matter whether you know what they look like. The "sense" of a person will do. You do *not* need to be on the phone with them, nor do you need their picture, a piece of their jewelry, a sample of their handwriting, or a lock of their hair.

Be with this person. Allow the vibrations of these frequencies to become larger and stronger. At times I'll bring in some of the work I teach in the advanced seminars, but it isn't necessary for this. It's simply something I like to do.

Be in this process as long as you like—whether it's for one minute or one hour. You may even choose to go further and enter into the "gap." Initially, be conscious of your intention, then let yourself enter.

Does the other person have to be aware of what you're doing? No.

I had a friend in southern Florida who called because his mother was in a hospital in northern Florida, about four or five hours' drive away from him. Apparently she had taken a turn for the worse, and the hospital had called to tell him that she wasn't expected to make it. They didn't really expect her to live long enough for him to make the drive up to see her. He phoned me in L.A. and asked if I would do a distance healing on her.

I'd never met my friend's mother, and she wasn't consciously available for me to ask her permission nor even to be aware of what I was going to do—but I agreed.

So I went into that *place*, and she and I met there. I allowed the sensations to course over and through me. Fifteen minutes later, I felt that the healing was complete. My friend phoned the next day and told me that his mother had had a complete turn for the better, totally surprising the hospital staff. She was released the following day. Her turnaround occurred while he was in his car, driving up to see her. It happened while she and I were together in the gap.

Was her recovery due to our interaction? I don't know. Are the reconnective frequencies moving at speeds faster than light? Quite probably— and with everything being light and light being everything, perhaps we should say faster than *visible* light. Are we operating at the negative space-time levels of people's higher dimensional components? Is what we're doing, then, organizing and supporting the molecular/cellular structures of the physical body? Maybe reorganizing it?

The concept of magnetoelectric realms and negative entropy potentially lend some intriguing insights into both reconnective distance healing and the reconnective frequencies and their interaction with self-healing and proximal healing.

Choice and Permission

> *"Karmageddon: It's like, when everybody is sending*
> *off all these really bad vibes, right? And then, like,*
> *the earth explodes, and it's like a serious bummer."*
> — The Washington Post

Choice and permission are two concepts that are somewhat intertwined. Not that everyone and everything aren't "one," anyway, it's just that these two ideas have an interesting relationship when it comes to healing. A discussion of them tends to bring up some fervent emotions in my seminars, so I often save the topic for just after lunch—in case a heavy meal has made any of the participants sleepy.

Let's start with *choice.* One of the biggest guilt trips that has been making the rounds for quite some time relates to this concept. I do not intend to do an exhaustive review here, but I do want to give you enough information to make a point.

Hang out at any New Age bookstore or gathering long enough and inevitably, as soon as a discussion turns to someone's faltering health, someone else will pipe in, generally with a *holier-than-thou* tone in their voice, and say, "Well, I wonder what they did to bring it on themselves." The others will then nod their heads in a practiced, all-knowing fashion.

We've all seen this. Now this poor person, whoever they are, already has enough going on without a group of NAGs (New Age Gossipers) attempting to make themselves feel superior at this person's expense. "Bob (or Mary or whoever) should simply choose to get well," the conversation continues. "Just look at what this is doing to their kids." The Spiritual One-upmanship is so thick you could cut it with a crystal wand.

If we were able to make our own choices as easily as we were able to select a shirt or a slice of pizza, I'd certainly choose to be happy, healthy, living in a loving relationship with a partner who fulfilled my every wish and need, and to be prosperous in the career of my choice. And, while I was at it, I'd choose to be incredibly good-looking (what the heck!). I know that a lot of you would choose some of these very same things. I also know that if there was a pill that could give this to us, we'd all be at our doctor's office first thing in the morning, standing in line for the prescription.

So why don't we all manifest these things in our lives to the degree we think we'd like? Because the part of us that does the choosing isn't the part of us that many would like to *think* does the choosing. It's not the conscious part of us that decides upon the blue shirt or the pepperoni pizza. It's the part of us that sees the big picture, the overview of our lives. It's the part of us that has the understanding that we're going through our lessons here on Earth and that our experiences are to be played out within certain parameters—those that we most likely agreed upon prior to incarnating this time around. Do I know this for a fact? No. Does it make sense? Yes.

So maybe Bob (or Mary) can't just order themselves up an instant helping of "good health." Maybe blaming them for that, *or for getting sick in the first place*, isn't really doing anyone a service. As more and more of us are able to view things from a larger perspective, there will be less pain inflicted on others by those of us who really want to mean well.

So, what does this have to do with asking for someone's permission prior to a healing?

Basically, asking permission of someone who has come to your office and is already lying on your table is, obviously—and politely put—redundant. (And, yes, I've actually seen healers do so.) Now, if you're already getting your back up, *go* back up and reread the previous few paragraphs on "choice," paying careful attention to the part about *who* it is that's doing the choosing—because this is the same part of you that's granting the permission.

Let's say that you have a beautiful five-year-old child. "Johnny" has been sick since he's been one and a half, and he lives in pain on a daily basis. His hair's falling out, and his medications make him nauseated. Most of his days are spent between his bedroom and his bathroom. He's precious, he's beautiful, he's stoic.

One day you get word of an amazing healer, a monk living in a cave in the Himalayas. You contact the monk and make arrangements to fly him in because Johnny's not strong enough to make the flight out of the country. You put up the monk in a nice hotel, and after a day's rest, you pick him up and bring him to your home. When he arrives, you lead him upstairs to Johnny's room. After a few minutes' worth of conversation, it's readily apparent that the monk and the boy have bonded. Now, with gravity and respect, the healer leans forward and says to your son, "Johnny, may I have your permission to give you a healing?" Johnny, who can't imagine life without pain—and therefore associates "healing" only with a longer life filled with more pain—thinks for a moment. Then, softly and somberly, he says, "No." Who do you want to strangle first—Johnny or the healer?

In all seriousness, Earthly informed consent isn't always *Informed* consent. Truly informed consent is more of a *misinformed* consent.

Johnny didn't give his permission because he couldn't see past his present situation. He based his decision on misinformation. His consent, or lack thereof, wasn't *informed;* it was *misinformed.* How many of us truly have all the answers? How many of us can see what our futures hold?

Much as some would have it appear otherwise, you can only *offer* a healing; you can't *inflict* a healing. Permission, therefore, is automatically requested as part of the act of offering. The healing, as it comes to fruition, is the permission being granted. So whether the person is a conscious recipient, such as someone who phones you for an appointment, or an individual who may not be able to make a conscious choice at the time, offering a healing, either verbally or in the silence of your own thought, is always appropriate. Both its acceptance and the form it takes are done with that person's highest good in mind.

What Is a Successful Healing?

What determines a successful healing? Is it someone who gets up out of a wheelchair and walks? Is it the disappearance of disease? Is it the restructuring and transformation of our DNA?

Or maybe life's the disease and death is the healing.

One day I received a call from an oncologist who asked if I would be able to see one of his patients. I said, "Of course." This woman wasn't able to leave the hospital, so I met her and her husband there, late in the evening. When I arrived, she was asleep, so I spoke with her husband for a little while, then began the session. Within a few moments, she opened her eyes. He introduced us, and throughout the duration of the session, the couple carried on a very animated and fun conversation. You could see the effects that the chemo and other long-term treatments had taken on her, yet you could also see the sparkle of beauty in her smile and in her eyes.

They were a young couple, probably in their 30s. When they spoke to one another, their eyes locked like two lovers who had just been reunited after a long separation. It was readily apparent that they enjoyed each other and that they were very much in love. She spoke, he listened; he spoke, she listened. They laughed and brought me into their conversation as if I were a long-time friend. They shared stories of different things they'd done together, and told me about their trips and of people in their lives.

All of a sudden, the woman was craving ice cream—three different kinds! I had already been at the hospital far later than I had planned, but I offered to stay longer while her husband went for food. As he was about to leave, she decided that cheesecake would also be nice. It was 11:00 P.M., yet nothing could have made the man happier than to find all these items and bring them back to his wife. He promised he'd return quickly, although we all knew that by the time he made it out of the hospital complex, found someplace that was open, and returned with everything, it would be a good 45 minutes. And it was. It was also one of the *longest* 45 minutes I'd experienced because, as the door closed behind him, she turned toward me and said, "I'm going to leave now."

I said, "You're *what?*" I knew what she meant, yet I couldn't believe what I was hearing.

"I'm going to leave now," she repeated.

"Now?" I asked.

She nodded.

I was somewhat in shock. The woman's demeanor and expression left no room for misinterpretation. She was telling me that she was planning to die, and planning to die *right then.* She had sent her husband on the food-run to assure that he wouldn't be present when she passed.

"Oh no, you're not," I told her.

I had no intention of his coming back with arms full of ice cream and cheesecake and finding me sitting next to his dead wife.

"I'm going to leave now," she repeated.

"You're going to stay right here until your husband gets back," I informed her in response to this third and most recent threat, glancing at the clock and noticing how slowly time seemed to be moving. The point was, I had no doubt that she could have "left" at that very moment. The only way to prevent this from happening was to keep her in conversation. I knew that once I let her stop talking, she was going to let go and cross over.

I told the woman that if she was making this decision to go, her husband would want the opportunity to say good-bye. I was keeping her thought processes engaged, and that was good. At this point, I'd have grabbed a ukelele and played *Tiptoe Through the Tulips* if I thought it would keep her alive until he came back. We talked. She "stayed."

About 45 minutes later, her husband returned. There was no mention of her "leaving." They resumed normal conversation as if nothing had occurred. My heart was still pounding as the woman ate her ice cream. They offered me some. I . . . wasn't very hungry. I said my good-nights and made a quick departure.

The husband called the next day to let me know that she had passed.

I already knew. He told me then that she had been asleep and/or mostly incoherent for close to two months prior to our visit. This was the first time that she had been lucid for more than a minute or so. He thanked me for giving him back his wife for that one final evening.

Who had the healing, and what was it? Well, they *each* had a healing. He needed, after two months, to see his wife one last time, to say good-bye and let go. She needed to see him again and know that he would be okay if she left. They each received their gift.

People die. We move on. It's part of our cosmic experience to recycle.

When someone does cross over, it doesn't mean that they didn't have a healing. Their healing may very well have been the ease with which you allowed them to have their transition, the peace they received through your visit to accept and let go—and that chance to smile and say "I love you" to someone who needed to hear it—one last time.

So don't interpret, don't analyze. Just be. And know that you carry the gift of healing—in whatever form that may take.

⨐ ⨐ ⨐

≫ CLOSING THOUGHTS ≪

The Wonder of It All

In this book, we've discussed healing as discovery, healing as theory, and healing as practice. But in closing, there's one aspect I want to emphasize: healing as *miracle*. By "miracle," I mean exactly that—a wondrous event manifesting a supernatural act of God. Of course, in a universe of quarks and black holes and 11 dimensions, *supernatural* doesn't mean what it used to. Then again, neither does *God*.

Still, the sense of awe and wonder that comes when the "impossible" occurs never diminishes. You see, when you facilitate these energies, you're not just assisting one person's healing—you're helping usher in a transformation of a magnitude heretofore unknown.

People ask me if *everyone* has the ability to carry these frequencies and become a healer. My answer is, "Yes. Everyone can reach this level, but eyes are blind. It is only a few who dare to open their eyes . . . and often those who do are blinded by what they see."

This, to me, is what Deepak Chopra meant when he told me to "remain childlike." Everything amazes children; they see the world as a brand-new adventure every day. Without our limited context to put things in, they are not *blinded* by *anything* they see. Without being taught fear, they do not limit with "shoulds," "shouldn'ts," obligatory ritual, or seriousness. It's all a part of the wondrous universe they have come to inhabit.

I feel that same excitement every day. Every time I do this work, I experience it with a sense of newness and discovery, as if it were my very first time. Because, with any particular person, it *is* the very first time. I know that you will feel this way, too. You're bringing into existence light and information that uniquely becomes the two (actually, the Three, including God) of you.

When this *gift* first presented itself, I was already a doctor with a very large practice. Therefore, I presumed that this gift was about healing. I knew that something *very big* was happening, and I called it *healing* because I thought it *was* about healing (in an expanded doctor/patient/miracle sense of the word)—and because I *wanted* it to be about healing.

I now see that, from the beginning, it was my *intention* for this gift to be about healing. I wanted to *understand* it, to *classify* it—and most likely later, to *direct* and *"enhance"* it. Healing was the context within which I practiced, and the context within which lay the hidden limitations I imposed upon The Reconnection. These weren't intentional limitations; they were simply those brought about by my inability to see further, to recognize from the very beginning that this was about something much larger.

What I've come to recognize is that this is healing in a very different sense than what we have been taught to perceive, understand, or even believe or accept. This healing is about an evolutionary process brought into existence through *co-creation* at the highest vibrational interaction with the Universe. I have come to believe that it is truly about the restructuring of our DNA, even though I was hesitant to say this at first. When we move into the transsensory—or *transcendsory*—(meaning beyond our basic five senses), we move into a realm of co-existence with an energy and presence beyond what we have known before.

My intention may well have redirected some of this to fit the earlier scope of my beliefs and understanding. And, while I teach that we are to get out of the way, to not direct or even intend the form the healing is to take, I realize that I had been *in* the way from the moment I made the decision that this was only about doctor/patient/miracle healing.

The problem wasn't that I had intention—it was the *specificity* of the intention. I took my wide-eyed state of *expectancy* and, through the specificity of my desires and intentions, viewed it through the narrowest scope of *expectation.*

Deepak Chopra, author of what I consider to be one of the most important books any of us can read, *The Seven Spiritual Laws of Success,* explains that one of the *Laws of Intention and Desire* is to "relinquish your attachment to the outcome. This means giving up your rigid attachment to a specific result and living in the wisdom of uncertainty." To a degree, many of us do this now. I did so to the extent that I relinquished my attachment to the outcome *of the healings.* I didn't, however, relinquish my attachment to the outcome *being* a healing; therefore, I limited my own experience.

You and I may now move forward. To do so, we must stay conscious of our intentions, those so subtly ingrained that they hover for the most part just below our conscious radar. When they "bleep" in on our screen, it is our responsibility to examine them. Our hidden intentions affect the direction we take, often more strongly than our conscious intentions, because we are not sufficiently aware of them to bring them to the light of examination. If we don't know we have the fear, we don't know to face it.

Through the information imparted in this book, you are undergoing your own evolutionary transition. You are now able to listen and hear with a different sense; to see with a new vision. You have learned to feel that which others have not yet felt. As you learned to experience this new awareness, you moved into your existence as a transcendsory being.

Now, when those who come to you for sessions hear *when there is nothing audible to others,* smell *when they have no physical sense of smell,* see *when their eyes are closed,* and feel *when, to the onlooker, there would be nothing to cause the feeling*—you know that you are escorting them into *their* new transcendsory level of existence as well. And it's as exciting each time as it was when you discovered it for yourself.

What you are doing is bringing light and information onto the planet—and where there is light and information, there can be no darkness. Through this light and information, among other things, come transformation and healing.

Healing is not the "how" or "why"—nor is it a recipe. It is a state of *being.*

So, with your fear, step into the light and information. Love *becomes* it. Then *it* becomes *love*—and *it* is the healer. *You* are at once the observer and the observed, the lover and the loved, the healer and the healed.

Become one with the other person, then heal *yourself.* In healing yourself, you heal others. And in healing others, you heal yourself.

Reconnect. Heal others; heal yourself.

Some things are difficult to explain; miracles speak for themselves.

➴ ➴ ➴

Read This Book
<u>Three</u> Times.

You haven't really read *The Reconnection* once until you've read it three times.

No matter how many times you've read *The Reconnection: Heal Others, Heal Yourself,* you'll discover that there's more to be found in each reading. You may have already discovered that it's written on an infinite number of levels. Not necessarily intentionally, and definitely not by my conscious design, yet there it is, just the same. Each time you read *The Reconnection,* you will find more insight—*light and information*—awaiting you. So, *read it again.* Then read it *again. Write* in it. *Highlight* it. *Review* it. There's more to be discovered. A *lot* more.

SHARE THE Reconnection.

Many of you who read *The Reconnection* will want to share what's in this book. As we all know, the gift of healing is one of the highest gifts we can offer. For those of us who are into consciousness, enlightenment, and evolution, for pretty much every one of us who loves our family and friends, *The Reconnection* is probably one of the most exciting and valuable gifts to give and receive. A gift of presence. So whether you choose to share your copy or give someone their very own, know that *what you are doing is Reconnecting "strands." What you are doing is Reconnecting "strings." What you are doing is bringing "light" and "information" onto the planet.*

ABOUT THE AUTHOR

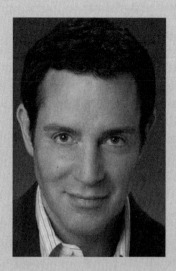

Dr Eric Pearl walked away from one of the most successful chiropractic practices in Los Angeles when he and others started witnessing miraculous healings. Since that time, he has committed himself to imparting the light and information of the Reconnective Healing process through extensive lectures and seminars about 'The Reconnection'.

Dr Pearl has appeared on countless television programs in the United States and around the world. He has also spoken by invitation at the United Nations, has presented to a full house at Madison Square Garden, and his seminars have been featured in various publications, including the *New York Times*.

www.TheReconnection.com

For Your Protection

This book will introduce you to information that can assist you in your initial interactions with Reconnective Healing. However, reading this book by itself will not make you a Reconnective Healing Practitioner or Reconnection Practitioner, allow you to teach Reconnective Healing® or The Reconnection®, or allow you to represent yourself to others as a Reconnective Healing Practitioner or Reconnection Practitioner or teacher of either or both. Successful completion of the seminars taught by Eric Pearl is a requirement in becoming a Reconnective Healing Practitoner or Reconnection Practitioner.

Presently Eric Pearl is the only authorized and qualified instructor teaching Reconnective Healing and The Reconnection. Eric is beginning to offer seminars to train instructors in Reconnective Healing and The Reconnection. Information on the Instructor Program seminars may be posted on Eric's Website and/or included in his brochures. You may also obtain this information by contacting The Reconnection at the email and phone numbers listed. You are required to have successfully completed the two basic weekend courses before progressing into training to become a Certified Practitioner, Teaching Assistant and Mentor, or to enter the Instructor Program. Other prerequisites may apply and may from time to time change.

For your protection, please contact us at info@TheReconnection.com or by phone at +1-323-960-0012 or 1-888-ERIC PEARL (1-888-374-2732) prior to attending any seminar that proposes to offer training in Reconnective Healing or The Reconnection taught by anyone other than Eric Pearl. We will let you know whether you are attending a seminar taught by a qualified instructor.

To find out more about the requirements for becoming a Reconnective Healing Practitioner, Reconnection Practitioner, Certified Practitioner, Teaching Assistant and Mentor, to enter into the Instructor Program or simply to remain a practitioner in good standing, please contact us at info@TheReconnection.com or by phone at +1-323-960-0012 or 1-888-ERIC PEARL (1-888-374-2732). We look forward to your comments and inquiries.

꩜ ꩜ ꩜

Contact Information for Dr. Eric Pearl and The Reconnection

Dr. Eric Pearl
c/o The Reconnection
P.O. Box 3600
Hollywood, CA 90078-3600
Website: **www.TheReconnection.com**
E-mail: **info@TheReconnection.com**

To attend a seminar or
to co-sponsor a seminar in your area, phone:
+1-323-960-0012
or
1-888-Eric Pearl (1-888-374-2732)
or e-mail
info@TheReconnection.com

For information on private sessions with a practitioner,
visit our Online Practitioner Directory at
www.TheReconnection.com
or phone
1-323-960-0012

Please send Dr. Pearl your healing stories that either
resulted from your reading this book, from a private session
with a practitioner, or from attending one of Dr. Pearl's seminars.
Please send them to the above mailing (postal) or e-mail addresses.
We look forward to hearing from you!

❧ NOTES ❧

❧ NOTES ❧

NOTES

NOTES

❧ NOTES ❧

NOTES

NOTES

We hope you enjoyed this Hay House book.
If you would like to receive a free catalogue featuring additional
Hay House books and products, or if you would like information
about the Hay Foundation, please contact:

Hay House UK Ltd
292B Kensal Road • London W10 5BE
Tel: (44) 20 8962 1230; Fax: (44) 20 8962 1239
www.hayhouse.co.uk

***

Published and distributed in the United States of America by:
Hay House, Inc. • PO Box 5100 • Carlsbad, CA 92018-5100
Tel: (1) 760 431 7695 or (1) 800 654 5126;
Fax: (1) 760 431 6948 or (1) 800 650 5115
www.hayhouse.com

***

Published and distributed in Australia by:
Hay House Australia Ltd • 18/36 Ralph Street • Alexandria, NSW 2015
Tel: (61) 2 9669 4299, Fax: (61) 2 9669 4144
www.hayhouse.com.au

***

Published and distributed in the Republic of South Africa by:
Hay House SA (Pty) Ltd • PO Box 990 • Witkoppen 2068
Tel/Fax: (27) 11 467 8904
www.hayhouse.co.za

***

Published and distributed in India by:
Hay House Publishers India • Muskaan Complex • Plot No.3
B-2• Vasant Kunj • New Delhi - 110 070
Tel: (91) 11 41761620; Fax: (91) 11 41761630
www.hayhouse.co.in

***

Distributed in Canada by:
Raincoast • 9050 Shaughnessy St • Vancouver, BC V6P 6E5
Tel: (1) 604 323 7100
Fax: (1) 604 323 2600

***

Sign up via the Hay House UK website to receive the Hay House
online newsletter and stay informed about what's going on with your
favourite authors. You'll receive bimonthly announcements
about discounts and offers, special events, product highlights,
free excerpts, giveaways, and more!
www.hayhouse.co.uk

JOIN THE HAY HOUSE FAMILY

As the leading self-help, mind, body and spirit publisher in the UK, we'd like to welcome you to our family so that you can enjoy all the benefits our website has to offer.

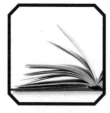

EXTRACTS from a selection of your favourite author titles

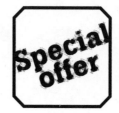

COMPETITIONS, PRIZES & SPECIAL OFFERS Win extracts, money off, downloads and so much more

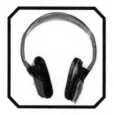

LISTEN to a range of radio interviews and our latest audio publications

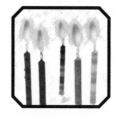

CELEBRATE YOUR BIRTHDAY An inspiring gift will be sent your way

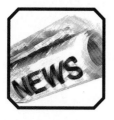

LATEST NEWS Keep up with the latest news from and about our authors

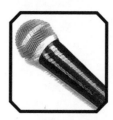

ATTEND OUR AUTHOR EVENTS Be the first to hear about our author events

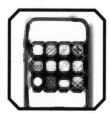

iPHONE APPS Download your favourite app for your iPhone

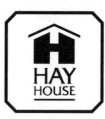

HAY HOUSE INFORMATION Ask us anything, all enquiries answered

join us online at **www.hayhouse.co.uk**

292B Kensal Road, London W10 5BE
T: 020 8962 1230 E: info@hayhouse.co.uk